# OBSERVATION AND INFERENCE

*An Introduction to the Methods of Epidemiology*

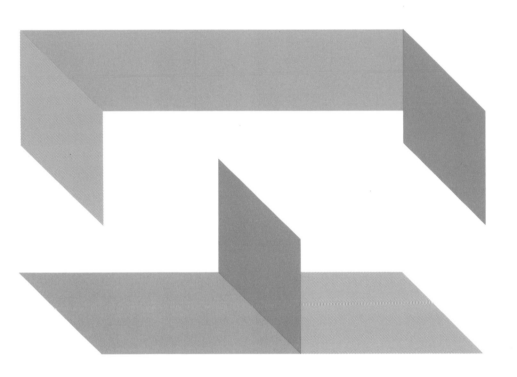

Alexander M. Walker

# OBSERVATION AND INFERENCE
## *An Introduction to the Methods of Epidemiology*

**Alexander M. Walker, MD, DrPH**

Epidemiology Resources Inc.

1991

# OBSERVATION AND INFERENCE

*An Introduction to the Methods of Epidemiology*

Epidemiology Resources Inc.
One Newton Executive Park
Newton Lower Falls, MA 02162
Telephone (617) 244-1200


**Library of Congress Cataloging-in-Publication Data:**

Walker, Alexander Muir
    Observation and inference : an introduction to the methods of epidemiology / Alexander M. Walker.
        p.        cm.
    Includes index.
    ISBN 0-917227-07-7
    1. Epidemiology--Methodology.    I. Title.
    [DNLM: 1. Epidemiologic Methods.    WA 105 W1770]
RA652.4.W35    1991
614.4--dc20
DNLM/DLC
for Library of Congress

Printed in the United States of America

*For Trish*

# Preface

"You've got a 20 percent chance of having another infarction this year," says the doctor, and you live an uneventful 12 months. Was the doctor right? You have an infarction. Was he wrong?

A statement of risk for an individual assumes that the individual belongs to a class and that a known fraction of the class's members possess a feature (such as "infarction within a year"). Obese, non-diabetic, white, 50 year old men experiencing an uncomplicated second myocardial infarction have a 20 percent chance of another infarction within 12 months. Advice to a patient about his risk is a double statement of class membership and of a characteristic of the class. If the class membership is wrong (do you *know* that he's not diabetic?), the problem is one of misclassification. If the fraction is wrong, then the problem concerns measurements that are the core of epidemiology.

The embodiment of a class is a population. Epidemiologists study the occurrence of disease in human populations.

Like bench scientists, epidemiologists have their share of false starts, wrong premises, and tentative approximations to a truth. Unlike their laboratory colleagues, epidemiologists operate under public scrutiny. Physicians, regulators, manufacturers and the judiciary are confronted daily with epidemiologic observations that may constitute the only relevant data on questions of health. The purpose of this text is to serve both the scrutinizers and the practicing epidemiologist as a guide.

There are several kinds of reading that I had in mind in preparing the manuscript. On the briefest level, it is possible to scan the definitions alone; these are marked by a bold faced lead term followed by italic descriptive text. A second level would comprise all the text apart from the statistical development of Chapters 6, 7, and 8. I hope that most readers will take on the more mathematical material as well. Epidemiology is comprehensible without algebra, but those who are not "numerate" need to keep in mind that there is a large and enjoyable area of epidemiologic science that they are unready to explore.

# Contents

# 1

# Disease Frequency

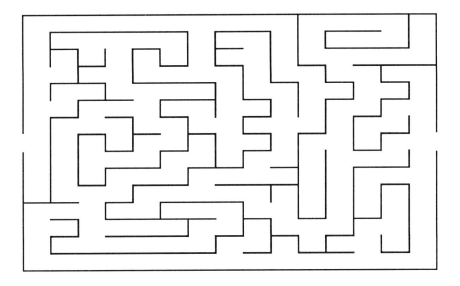

The building blocks of epidemiology are rooted in experience: we "know" what disease is, we know what a toxic exposure might be, and we can count noses. The language of epidemiology is full of terms from everyday speech, terms that have both formal meanings and all the connotations that the same words carry in general use. The associations with day-to-day ideas can be helpful in spirit, but they can be misleading in particulars. The purpose of this first chapter is therefore to define and illustrate, with an emphasis on the components of observation in a single population. Subsequent chapters will deal with comparisons, methods for structuring observation, and the barriers that stand between observation and inference.

## Cross-Sectional Measures

The simplest population measure of disease burden is prevalence.

**Prevalence.** *The prevalence of a characteristic in a population is the fraction of individuals in the population who possess the characteristic.*

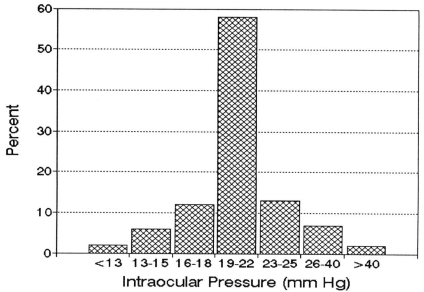

**Figure 1.1** The prevalence of intraocular pressure readings in diabetics attending the Joslin Clinic in 1935

A prevalence is a status report. Since most characteristics of any interest vary with time as well as across populations, any mention of a prevalence ought to be accompanied by a specification of whom and of when. Figure 1.1 graphs the prevalence of various levels of intraocular pressure (IOP) among 2,002 diabetics over the age of 20 seen at the Joslin Clinic (in Boston) in the years 1925 through 1934.[1] Most of the readings summarized in Figure 1.1 were normal, and the data were interpreted as indicating that diabetics do not as a group suffer from intraocular hypertension. In the non-diabetic population, however, about five percent of adults have IOPs higher than 22 millimeters of mercury (mm Hg). On the basis of Figure 1.1, the

---

1. Waite JH, Beetham WP. N Engl J Med 1935;212:367-369

prevalence of IOPs greater than 22 mm Hg appears to have been about 20 percent. The authors' opinion notwithstanding, diabetics at the Joslin Clinic had an excess prevalence of intraocular hypertension.

**Table 1.1** Use of NSAIDs, acetaminophen, and antacids two years prior to a first prescription for cimetidine

|  | Subsequent Users of Cimetidine N = 1327 | Age-Matched Subsequent Non-Users N = 5308 |
|---|---|---|
| Any NSAID | 338 (25%) | 907 (17%) |
| Acetaminophen | 382 (29%) | 906 (17%) |
| Antacids | 521 (39%) | 889 (17%) |

Prevalence can be of special usefulness in assessing the disease burden of a community and in projecting demands for medical services. The annual cost, *per capita* of the general population, of caring for persons with AIDS can be estimated by multiplying the prevalence of AIDS by $25,000.

Table 1.1 gives the prevalence of use of several analgesics in persons aged 65 and older in two populations.[2] The first population consisted of people who would be diagnosed two years later as having significant peptic ulcer disease (indicated by the receipt of a first prescription for the anti-ulcer drug cimetidine[3]), the second population consisted of persons of similar age and sex who would have no such diagnosis. Are these prevalences compatible with the idea that there is no relation between the use of these drugs and peptic ulcer disease (PUD)? Even without formal tests of statistical significance, it seems scarcely credible that the differences in Table 1.1 could be ascribable to chance. One possibility is that the drugs considered *cause* PUD. Alternatively, it may be that the drugs are being used to treat early symptoms of PUD, even in advance of a

2. The study from which these data are drawn is described in: Hernandez Avila M, Walker AM, Romieu I, et al. Choice of nonsteroidal anti-inflammatory drug in persons treated for dyspepsia. Lancet 1988;ii:556-9

3. At present, use of cimetidine would be a very nonspecific indicator of peptic ulcer disease. In the late 1970s, when the data of Table 1.1 were collected, the connection was thought to be much closer.

specific diagnosis. The connection is evident in the case of antacids, but holds for the analgesics (nonsteroidal anti-inflammatory drugs -- "NSAIDs" -- and acetaminophen) as well. Persons with early, undiagnosed PUD may have nonspecific pains that are incorrectly diagnosed as arthritic, for which analgesics are prescribed. This supposition is strengthened particularly by the increased use of acetaminophen, for which (unlike the NSAIDs) there is little non-epidemiologic evidence of gastrointestinal toxicity.

**Measures that Incorporate Fixed Intervals of Time**

Prevalence does not capture the concept of elapsed time, and it offers no information about *transitions* between states of health and disease. For the resource planner, knowing the prevalent number of ill people may be enough, but for both the patient and the physician, the transition from one health state to another is a key event.

One way to examine transition probabilities is to string together a series of prevalences over time. Assuming that the entire population remains under observation, the change between prevalences at successive times is a measure of the net rate of transition into the morbid state. If more people get sick than get well, then the prevalence rises. If the state is irreversible, then the difference in successive prevalences is related to the number of new or *incident* cases.

**Incident.** *A case of disease is said to be "incident" at the moment at which the disease manifests signs or symptoms. Incident cases are newly occurring cases.*

The definition of an incident case depends on the current technical ability to recognize disease. The distinction of times of onset is important, but often approximate, particularly in the case of chronic diseases. Rather than wait for an unimpeachable definition of disease onset, most investigators proceed with the understanding that the operative definition may change, and that conclusions may have to be revised.

Even with reversible conditions, prevalences can be calculated at successive points in time as if the condition were irreversible. That is, people go from the state "has never suffered event X" to the state "has suffered event X at some time in the past." In the absence of loss to follow-up among the study subjects, prevalences obtained by this convention are measures of the *cumulative incidence.*[4]

**Cumulative incidence.** *The cumulative incidence from time $t_0$ to time $t_1$ for event X is the prevalence of "history of X" at time $t_1$ among all those persons who began observation at time $t_0$ and did not possess a "history of X" at time $t_0$.*

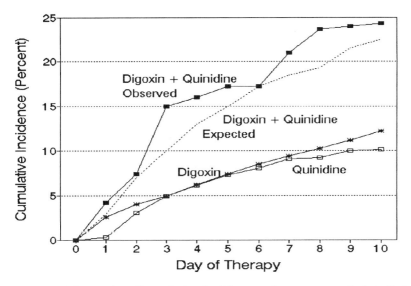

**Figure 1.2** Cumulative incidence of symptoms of digitalis intoxication in patients receiving digoxin and/or quinidine

Figure 1.2[5] gives the cumulative incidence of signs and symptoms of digitalis intoxication in hospitalized patients receiving digoxin

4. Other terms for cumulative incidence include "incidence proportion" and "risk." The former provides a neat linguistic tie to "incidence rate," defined later; the latter emphasizes the connection to probability of disease; the principal drawback of the term "risk" is that the same word can be used to denote both observed events and the underlying forces of morbidity that generated the events.

5. Walker AM, Cody RJ, Greenblatt DJ, Jick H. Drug toxicity in patients receiving digoxin and quinidine. Am Heart J 1983;105:1025-8

alone and digoxin plus quinidine (instituted on Day 0). Also shown are the cumulative incidences of clinically similar events in patients receiving quinidine alone, and the sum of the curves for digoxin alone and quinidine alone. Administration of quinidine to patients receiving digoxin increases serum digoxin levels through displacement of digoxin from albumin and from tissue binding sites, and the expectation was that concurrent therapy would increase the risk for digoxin side effects. The observed digoxin-with-quinidine curve is higher than the curves for the drugs separately, but only slightly above the sum of the two.[6] Elevated blood levels notwithstanding, there is little evidence here for a clinical effect attributable specifically to the concurrent administration of digoxin and quinidine.

The cumulative incidence over each of the one-day intervals of Figure 1.2 might be referred to as a "daily cumulative incidence," and could be calculated as each day's number of incident cases divided by the number of persons who had not yet developed digitalis intoxication at the beginning of the day. The curve labeled "daily incidence" in Figure 1.3 presents the daily cumulative incidence of bleeding in patients receiving heparin therapy.[7]

Complementary to the cumulative incidence is the measure called *survival*.

**Survival** *is the complement of disease occurrence over a time interval. The observed survival is 1 minus the cumulative incidence of disease.*

Survivals in successive time periods can be multiplied together to obtain a cumulative survival. The cumulative incidence curves of

---

6. The method of comparison illustrated in Figure 1.2 is valid for the data shown, but should be generalized only with some caution because the addition of curves to give the digoxin-plus-quinidine "expected" curve overstates the expectation. First, from elementary probability theory, the combination of $P_D$, the probability of an adverse reaction as a result of digoxin, and $P_Q$, the corresponding probability for quinidine, to form $P_{D+Q}$, should not be $P_D + P_Q$ but rather $1-(1-P_D)(1-P_Q)$. Second, if there is any background probability of occurrence of something that might be misdiagnosed as digitalis toxicity, i.e. if signs or symptoms consistent with digitalis intoxication can be expected to occur in people receiving neither digitalis nor quinidine, then that background probability, $P_0$, has been counted twice when the curves are added. The true expected cumulative incidence curves would be given by $P_{D+Q+0} = 1-(1-P_D)(1-P_Q)(1-P_0)$, where the Ps refer to the probabilities uniquely associated with digoxin, quinidine, and background. In the present example, in which the component probabilities are not large, the true expected curve is close to the simple approximation graphed in Figure 1.2.

7. Walker AM, Jick H. Predictors of bleeding during heparin therapy. JAMA 1980;244:1209-1212

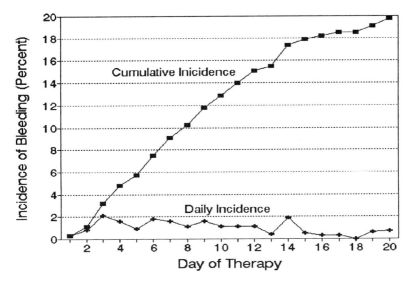

**Figure 1.3** Cumulative incidence and daily incidence of bleeding in patients receiving heparin

Figures 1.2 and 1.3 were derived by calculating daily survivals, multiplying these to arrive at cumulative survivals, and subtracting the result from 1.

**Measures for Variable Observation Times**

The definition of cumulative incidence assumes an opportunity to observe a group of persons from beginning to end of a time interval. More commonly, individuals possess characteristics that define their class membership for variable periods of time. The occurrence of disease is then measured not over a fixed interval, but over whatever intervals are eligible for observation from each person under study. The intervals are collectively called the *person time* of observation of a population.

**Person time** *is the time during which a single individual meets all the definitions for inclusion in a study, and during which any disease event occurring in the individual would be known. The person time of observation in a population is the sum of the person times contributed by all the members of the population.*

There are three equivalent methods for calculating the person time of observation of a population under study.

(1) For each person, identify the amount of time contributed to the group's observation, then sum the times of the individual persons to get person time.

(2) Multiply the number of persons under observation by the average duration of observation per person.

(3) Multiply the length of the period of observation by the average number of persons under observation during the period.

Unlike "persons," who are discrete and easily imagined, "person time" is a continuous quantity that proves difficult for most people to intuit. To visualize person time, think of a very small period of a person's experience, such as a day or an hour, as a discrete unit of observation. Each study subject contributes some number of units to a grand pool of observation.

A measure of disease frequency can be obtained by dividing the number of events that are observed among eligible population members by the total person time of observation.

**Incidence rate.** *The incidence rate of an event in a pool of person time is the number of events observed divided by the amount of person time observed.*

The general method of calculating an incidence rate in a specified population group during a given period of time has three parts:

(1) sum the number of cases that occur among members of the population during the time period in question;

(2) calculate the amount of person time of observation in the population for the time period;

(3) divide the number of cases by the person time of observation.

An incidence rate can be thought of as the fraction becoming ill, adjusted for length of follow-up. To see this algebraically, look at the second method for obtaining the person time of observation. With a little rearrangement, the procedure for calculating the incidence rate could be laid out as follows: divide the number of cases by the number of people observed to get the fraction becoming ill; next divide the fraction becoming ill by the average duration of observation to obtain the incidence rate.

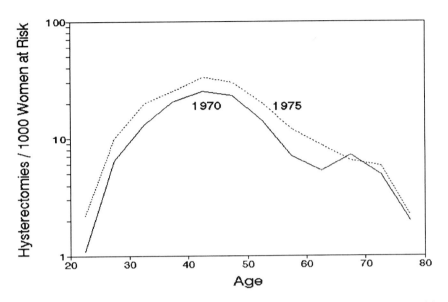

**Figure 1.4** Incidence rate of hysterectomy among women with an intact uterus, by United States Census Region, 1970

To justify an incidence rate calculation as a sensible procedure the analyst has to assume that the incidence rate is nearly constant throughout the pool of person time observed. If the incidence rate appears to vary over calendar time or within subgroups of a population of interest, then the time period of observation and the population must be split into subcategories, within which the assumption of constancy nearly holds. A series of appropriately labeled rates for the categories of person time, presented in tabular or graphic form, then serves to characterize the disease process in the population.

Figure 1.4 shows the incidence rate of hysterectomy per 1000 woman years at risk for women of various ages in the United States in 1970 and 1975.[8] The person times of observation were obtained using the third person-time method above. The rate was calculated for each age group in each of the two calendar years by estimating the number of women who had a uterus (the population at risk),

8. Walker AM, Jick H. Temporal and regional variation in hysterectomy rates in the United States, 1970-1975. Am J Epidemiol 1979;110:41-6

multiplying that figure by one year (yielding woman years at risk in 1970 or 1975), and dividing the resulting number into an estimate of the number of hysterectomies performed.

In 1970, hysterectomy rates in the 65-69 year age group were higher than those in the immediately young or older age groups. One interpretation of the 1970 curve in Figure 1.4 is that there is a discontinuity at age 65 in what should properly be a picture more like that seen five years later, a smooth curve with a single peak at 40-44 years. In this light, the high value among women in their late 60s in 1970 is just the leading figure in an elevation of the whole post-65 year portion of the age-incidence curve. Medicare, the U.S. government's program of payment for medical care to the elderly, was introduced in 1967. According to cynics observing the U.S. medical scene in the early 1970s, the two principal indications for hysterectomy at the time were a uterus and the ability to pay. The secondary peak in 1970 may have represented "catch-up" procedures in patients who had newly acquired the second indication.

Some characteristics of the measures of disease presented so far are listed in Table 1.2 at the end of this chapter. The information below the solid line refers to material presented in later chapters, but is included here for reference.

### Duration of Disease

The relation between the incidence rate of a disease and its prevalence involves the *duration* of disease.

**Duration.** *The duration of an illness is the length of the time interval that elapses from first manifestation of disease until complete resolution. For an irreversible disease process, duration is the length of the interval from first manifestation to death.*

A disease with a long duration may have a relatively high prevalence even if the disease has a low incidence. Multiple sclerosis (MS) has an overall incidence rate in the northern part of the United States of around 3 cases per 100,000 person years, less than one-tenth the incidence of cancer of lung, which is about 40 cases per 100,000 person years. Yet the prevalence of MS is much higher than that of cancer of the lung. The prevalence of MS is about 75 cases per 100,000 persons, versus about 40 cases per 100,000 persons for lung cancer. The MS prevalence is actually quite close to that of strep-tococcal pharyngitis, a commonly occurring disease (the incidence rate is on the order of 10,000 cases per 100,000 person years) that has a short duration. The discrepancy among the incidence rates and prevalences of these illnesses are accounted for by their different mean durations. The duration of MS is on the order of 25 years, that of lung cancer one year, and of symptomatic strep throat three days.

The interplay between the epidemiologic features of disease has a straightforward algebraic expression. When the prevalence is less than 10 percent (10,000 cases per 100,000 persons), the steady state relation between prevalence $(Pr)$, incidence rate $(IR)$, and mean duration $\overline{D}$ is

$$Pr = (IR)\overline{D}$$

The qualifier "steady state" imposes a number of strong restrictions on this relation. Newborns and immigrants (all healthy) must balance exactly the number without disease who die or emigrate, the number of diseased persons who immigrate must equal the number of diseased persons who emigrate, and the number of persons who become diseased per unit time must exactly equal the number of disease terminations, which may occur through a return to health or through death.

Although no free-living population is likely to meet the steady state criteria, the qualitative relation embodied in the preceding equation applies widely. A study of HLA types (a class of genetic markers) among children with acute lymphocytic leukemia (ALL) who attended an oncology clinic found that the prevalence of type A2 was higher than that in the general population.[9] The observation raised considerable interest, implying as it did that susceptibility to acute leukemia might be mediated by genetic factors. A follow-up study of a series of newly diagnosed leukemics found identical prevalences of the "high risk" type A2 in patients and in the general population.[10] The discordance between the two findings was due to an effect of HLA type on the mean duration of ALL. Far from being at high risk of ALL, children with HLA type A2 were at no

---

9. Rogentine GN, Yankee RA, Gart JJ, et al. HLA antigens and disease: acute lymphocytic leukemia. J Clin Invest 1972;51:2420-8. I am grateful to Philip Cole for pointing out this example in his chapter of introduction to Volume 1 of Statistical Methods in Cancer Research, The Analysis of Case-Control Studies, by N.E. Breslow and N.E. Day, International Agency for Research on Cancer, Lyon, 1980.

10. Rogentine GN, Trapani RJ, Yankee RA, Henderson ES. HLA antigens and acute lymphocytic leukemia: the nature of the association. Tissue Antigens 1973;3:470-6

increased risk, responded better to chemotherapy, had longer survivals, and were therefore overrepresented in the (prevalent) clinic population. The lesson is that if you want to study the determinants of incidence rate, you need incident rather than prevalent cases of disease.

A more general relation between prevalence, incidence rate, and duration, which holds for any prevalence, can be derived by observing that (a) if the total population size is $N$ then the population at risk for becoming diseased is $(1-Pr)N$ and the population at risk for leaving the diseased state is $PrN$, and (b) the rate of leaving the diseased state equals the reciprocal of the mean duration of the diseased state. The equation to be solved becomes "number entering diseased state in time interval $\Delta t$ = number leaving diseased state in $\Delta t$." That is

$$IR(1 - Pr)N\Delta t = \frac{1}{D} Pr N\Delta t$$

From which

$$\frac{Pr}{1 - Pr} = (IR)\overline{D}$$

**Table 1.2**
Measures of Disease Occurrence

| Measure | Prevalence | Cumulative incidence | Survival | Incidence rate |
|---|---|---|---|---|
| Incorporation of time | None | Specified follow-up | Specified follow-up | Incremental |
| Dimension | Cases per population | Cases per population after specified time | Nondiseased per population after specified time | Cases per population per unit time |
| Minimum Value | 0 | 0 | 0 | 0 |
| Maximum value | 1 | 1 | 1 | infinity |
| Parameter | Probability | Probability | Probability | Hazard |
| Probability Distribution | Binomial | Binomial | Binomial | Poisson |
| Variance | $\dfrac{Pr(1-Pr)}{N}$ | $\dfrac{CI(1-CI)}{N}$ | $\dfrac{S(1-S)}{N}$ | $\dfrac{IR}{P}$ |

# 2

# Comparisons

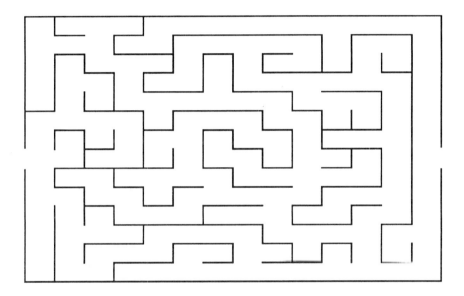

"A causes B." Scientists may mean that there is a regular temporal sequence of A then B, mediated by a physical mechanism that leads from one to the other. Even such a simple definition leaves room for ambiguity. A researcher who had studied the fates of insulation workers concluded that "All workers who have been heavily exposed to asbestos are certain to die of asbestos-related disease, unless they die of something else first." In striving to describe the effect of asbestos, the scientist had arrived at a tautology.

Estimates of "effect" in epidemiology are comparisons of measures such as those presented in the preceding chapter. Interpretation of the comparative measure as a statement about nature, however, demands further assumptions. The following three ideas provide a starting point.

**Generalizability.** *The physical processes that give rise to disease are largely similar in different individuals.*

**Individuals determine groups.** *Similar processes operating in different individuals give rise to predictable patterns of disease occurrence in groups.*[11]

**Groups reflect individuals.** *Patterns of disease occurrence in groups provide information about common physical processes operating within members of the group.*

With these ideas as their justification, epidemiologists derive mathematical expressions to summarize the differences between groups. The numerical relations among measured features of populations are the "measures of effect." They are a metaphor for disease processes within individuals. As with any metaphor, the image is powerful when it is precise and compact, and when it predicts that which was previously unseen.

Although there are infinitely many ways of joining even a pair of numbers, there are two that together have been used for almost all purposes of public health applications and etiologic research. These are *difference* measures and *ratio* measures.

**Difference Measures**

The *incidence rate difference* is a direct measure of the impact of an exposure.

**Incidence rate difference.** *The incidence rate difference is the difference between the incidence in an exposed population and that in an unexposed population.*

The incidence rate difference is also called simply the *rate difference*.[12] The term "incidence rate difference" is abbreviated as "*IRD*" or "*RD*."

---

11. Students of infectious disease and of population dynamics will point out that there are simple processes whose long term behavior is so unpredictable as to call this assumption into question. Repeated iteration of a recursive formula for the prevalence of a disease as a function of the prevalence at an earlier date,

$$Pr_{i+1} = kPr_i(1-Pr_i)$$

for k greater than about 2.72, yields this sort of long-run instability. The literature of disease transmission is replete with intractable mathematics that will be ignored here.

12. Or even the "risk difference" or the "attributable risk," though the latter two terms are misnomers.

Table 2.1 gives annual incidence rates of death from coronary heart disease (CHD) in men in two age categories.[13] The incidence rate difference between the heavier smokers and the nonsmoking men aged 55-64 is 468 deaths per 100,000 man years. For men aged 65-74 years, the difference is 695 deaths per 100,000 man years. The incidence rate difference associated with smoking is greater in the older age group.

**Table 2.1** Deaths from coronary heart disease per 100,000 man years

|  |  | Current smokers Cigarettes / day | |
| --- | --- | --- | --- |
| Age | Nonsmokers | 10 - 20 | 21 - 39 |
| 55-64 | 501 | 798 | 969 |
| 65-74 | 1,015 | 1,501 | 1,710 |

Comparable figures for lung cancer mortality are shown in Table 2.2. The incidence rate differences for lung cancer deaths are 360 and 640 cases per 100,000 man years for men aged 55-64 and 65-74 years respectively for the heavier smokers. The relations of cigarette smoking to coronary heart disease mortality and to lung cancer mortality are roughly the same, in the sense that nearly equal numbers of deaths from each cause would be avoided if smokers could be given the same mortality rates as nonsmokers.

**Table 2.2** Deaths from lung cancer per 100,000 man years

|  |  | Current smokers Cigarettes / day | |
| --- | --- | --- | --- |
| Age | Nonsmokers | 10 - 20 | 21 - 39 |
| 55-64 | 40 | 250 | 400 |
| 65-74 | 80 | 500 | 720 |

13. U.S. Public Health Service. The Health Consequences of Smoking. A Reference Edition: 1976. U.S. Department of Health, Education, and Welfare, Public Health Service, Centers for Disease Control, HEW Publication No. (CDC) 78-8357, 1976, pp 657 ff

Incidence rate differences give a measure of the burden of disease for exposed individuals. Since smoking principally affects those who smoke, the health implications of smoking for the general public are related to the numbers of smokers and nonsmokers in the population. The general population incidence associated with smoking is the incidence rate difference that would be obtained by comparing the mixed population of smokers and nonsmokers, as it naturally occurs, with a population composed purely of nonsmokers. This difference is the *population rate difference (PRD)*.[14]

**Population rate difference.** *The difference between an incidence rate in a population comprising both exposed and unexposed persons and the rate in a population comprising unexposed persons alone is the population rate difference.*

Algebraically,[15] the population rate difference can be shown to equal the incidence rate difference between exposed and unexposed, multiplied by the prevalence of the exposure in the population. Denote this last quantity by $f_1$, and let $IR_1$ and $IR_0$ be the incidence rates in exposed and unexposed, respectively. Then

$$PRD = f_1 ( IR_1 - IR_0 )$$

If forty percent of a male population aged 65-74 smoked 21-39 cigarettes a day, and nobody smoked more or less, then the *PRD* for coronary heart disease mortality would be calculable as follows:

$$f_1 = 0.4$$
$$IR_0 = 1,015$$

---

14. The PRD has been known as the "population attributable rate" and the "population attributable risk," both abbreviated PAR. The term "risk" is wrong in the present context. As discussed later, the word "attributable" is much stronger than warranted. Taken as technical jargon, the phrase was innocuous in an earlier time, but epidemiology so often enters into judicial and regulatory matters now that the misleading term needs to be corrected.

15. On the assumption that the members of a population have no individual risk that results from the smoking habits of their fellows, the incidence rate in the general population is the number of cases arising from exposed person time plus the number of cases arising from unexposed person time minus the number of cases that would have arisen had all the person time been subject to the rate of the unexposed, all divided by the total person time. Recognizing that the amount of exposed person time is $f_1P$ and that the amount of unexposed person time is $(1-f_1)P$, the definition of PRD becomes

$$PRD = \frac{IR_1 f_1 P + IR_0 (1 - f_1) P - IR_0 P}{P}$$

which simplifies to the expression given.

$$IR_1 = 1,710$$
$$PRD = 0.4 \; ( \; 1,710 - 1,015 \; )$$
$$= 278 \text{ cases per } 100,000 \text{ man years}$$

When there is more than one level of the exposure of interest, the defining equation is generalized to accommodate the prevalence of each exposure level, which is multiplied by the incidence rate difference appropriate to that level, and summed. Define $f_i$ as the prevalence of exposure level $i$ in the population, and let there be $N$ exposure levels. Then[16]

$$PRD = \sum_{i=1}^{N} f_i (IR_i - IR_0)$$

If thirty percent of a male population aged 65-74 smoked 10-20 cigarettes per day, and ten percent smoked 21-39 per day, then the PRD for coronary heart disease mortality would be calculable as follows:

$$f_1 = 0.3$$
$$f_2 = 0.1$$
$$IR_0 = 1,015$$
$$IR_1 = 1,501$$
$$IR_2 = 1,710$$
$$PRD = 0.3 \; ( \; 1,501 - 1,015 \; ) + 0.1 \; ( \; 1,710 - 1,015 \; )$$
$$= 215 \text{ cases per } 100,000 \text{ man years}$$

Since the PRD is a function of exposure prevalence as well as of the incidence of disease in exposed and unexposed, any presentation of the PRD should be accompanied by a specification of the population for which it was calculated. The PRD is zero when either the prevalence of exposure in the population is zero (i.e. when there is no exposure) or when the incidence rate difference is zero (when

---

16. The symbol immediately following the equality sign is a capital Greek letter sigma. It indicates that there should be a summation of terms whose form is given to the right of the sigma and that the terms should differ from one another by successive substitution of different values of one of the variables in the expression to the right. The i=1 below the sigma indicates that i is the variable to be successively changed, and that its first value should be 1. By convention, i should be successively increased by units of 1. The N above the sigma is the maximum value for i in the series; for unit increments in i, N is also the number of terms to be summed.

there is no effect of exposure). In the extreme case of all the population being exposed, the *PRD* equals the incidence rate difference.[17]

## Ratio Measures

Cigarette smoking is widely believed to be more strongly associated with lung cancer than it is with heart disease. The basis for this impression lies with the second major way of comparing incidence rates. The ratios of the mortality rates of coronary heart disease in smokers of 21-39 cigarettes per day to those in nonsmokers are given in Table 2.3, together with the corresponding ratios for mortality from lung cancer. Cigarette smoking raises lung cancer and CHD mortality rates by about the same amount, but the increase in lung cancer is over a much lower baseline. The result is that the relative mortality is much higher for lung cancer than for CHD.

**Table 2.3** Incidence rate ratios for deaths from lung cancer and coronary heart disease, comparing smokers (21-39 cigarettes/day) to nonsmokers

| Age | CHD | Lung cancer |
|-----|-----|-------------|
| 55-64 | 1.9 | 10 |
| 65-74 | 1.7 | 9 |

**Incidence rate ratio.** *The incidence rate ratio is the ratio of the incidence rate in an exposed population to that in an unexposed population.*

Incidence rate ratios (often called just *rate ratios*, and abbreviated as "*IRR*" or "*RR*") are heavily used in etiologic research. A large rate ratio is taken to indicate that the population characteristic being examined (here, smoking) is related to an important fraction of the disease in the exposed. The logic of this convention derives from the central role that the rate ratio plays in the answer to the question, "What fraction of the incidence rate (or cumulative incidence) in

---

17. The PRD could not be derived solely from the experience of a uniformly exposed population, since there would be no data on $IR_0$. It could nonetheless be estimated if there were an external estimate for $IR_0$, such as might be available from tables of vital statistics.

exposed persons could be eliminated, if the exposed could be given the same incidence rates as the unexposed?" The answer to this question is called the *relative excess incidence (REI)*.[18]

**Relative excess incidence.** *The relative excess incidence is the fraction of the disease burden among exposed that would not have occurred if the exposed had experienced the same incidence rate as the unexposed.*

The *REI* can be calculated from incidence rates or from cumulative incidences. The defining equation for the *REI* (written here in terms of incidence rates) is

$$REI = \frac{IR_1 - IR_0}{IR_1} = \frac{RR - 1}{RR}$$

Since the incidence rate ratio for lung cancer presented in Table 2.3 is 9.0 among older men, the fraction of the lung cancer disease burden among older, heavier smokers that is associated with smoking is

$$REI = \frac{9.0 - 1}{9.0} = 0.89$$

By contrast, the relative excess incidence for CHD mortality is

$$REI = \frac{1.7 - 1}{1.7} = 0.41$$

Nearly 90 percent of the lung cancer mortality rate in heavy smokers is associated with smoking, whereas less than half of the CHD mortality is so associated.

If an exposure affects the time course of onset of disease, the *REI* calculated on the basis of incidence rates may vary with time since exposure. By contrast, the *REI* based on cumulative incidences presents a single summary figure that integrates the full time of observation, and is insensitive to changes in times of onset. Note

---

18. The relative excess incidence has been referred to as the "etiologic fraction" (abbreviated EF) in a number of textbooks. Like "attributable," "etiologic," when prepended to "fraction," is a technical term whose meaning differs both from the common meaning and from that which epidemiologists themselves generally intend when they discuss etiology. Presentation of an "etiologic fraction" does not imply any special standard of proof of causation.

that an *REI* calculated on the basis of cumulative incidence becomes arbitrarily small as the reference cumulative incidence approaches one, whereas the *REI* based on incidence rates is unaffected. The choice between incidence rate and cumulative incidence as the basis of the *REI* calculation depends on the perspective of the user of the data. As a rule of thumb, use cumulative incidences when the time period over which disease occurs is such that there is no useful distinction between early and late onsets. Many studies of infectious disease have this property, as may studies of fetal loss.

## Mathematical Models of Incidence

Re-expressed as an equation or "model," the relation between the incidence rates in smokers and nonsmokers could be written as a function of the rate difference:

$$IR_1 = IR_0 + RD$$

or in terms of the rate ratio as

$$IR_1 = IR_0\,RR$$

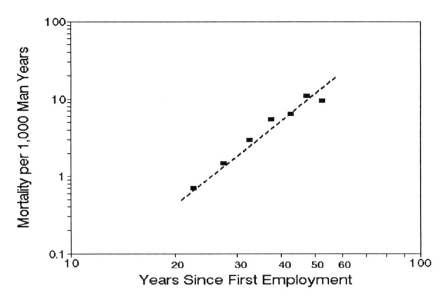

**Figure 2.1** Annual mortality from mesothelioma among North American insulation workers

Often one scale is clearly superior for the summary of a complex body of data. In the examples given above, a single rate ratio could pretty well describe overall effects of heavy smoking on CHD mortality. The ratio was nearly the same in the two age strata presented ($RR \approx 1.8$ ), whereas no single rate difference could even approximately describe both strata.

Effect relations that are too complex to summarize in a table can sometimes be described easily with a model of incidence. The annual incidence of mesothelioma in North American insulation workers employed before 1960 appears to be well described at any time t by the relation[19]

$$IR(t) = 0.00437 \ t^{3.2} \text{ cases } / \text{ 100,000 man years}$$

where $t$ is the elapsed time in years since an individual's first employment as an insulation worker. The relation is charted in Figure 2.1 on a log-log scale (that is with both axes scaled to the logarithm of the reported values).[20] Very similar relations have been seen in other populations occupationally exposed to asbestos, and in the resident population of Karain, Turkey, where fibrous minerals are omnipresent in exposed veins, in the dust on roads and in homes, and are used as the basic construction materials for all housing.[21] In Karain, $t_0$ is your day of birth.

Notice that there are two estimates of effect in the incidence model for mesothelioma among insulation workers. The first constant term (0.00437) gives the height of the curve; it reflects the intensity of asbestos exposure endured by the insulation workers. The second constant term (3.2) is an exponent to elapsed time, and presents a curvilinear "effect" of time on mesothelioma mortality.

---

19. Peto J, Seidman H, Selikoff IJ. Mesothelioma mortality in asbestos workers: Implications for models of carcinogenesis and risk assessment. Br J Cancer 1982;45:124-35

20. That Figure 2.1 should present a straight line follows immediately from the linear form of the incidence equation when logarithms are taken:

$$\ln(IR) = \ln(0.00437) + 3.2\ln(t)$$

The leading constant is an intercept. It gives the incidence at $\ln(t) = 0$, that is at t = 1 year.

21. Saracci R, Simonato L, Baris Y, Artvinli M, Skidmore J. The age-mortality curve of endemic pleural mesothelioma in Karain, Central Turkey. Br J Cancer 1982;45:147-9

## Group Comparisons and Individual Cause

Consider ten men who smoke cigarettes and among whom, apart from the effect of their workplace exposures, there would have been three lung cancer deaths at the ages of 55, 60, and 65.[22] Imagine that the effects of an inhaled workplace carcinogen were twofold: first, to induce changes in the composition of bronchial mucus so that particulate matter from cigarette smoke would be more effectively removed from the lungs; second and independently, to induce lung cancer through some direct effect on lung tissue. Imagine further that the net result of the opposing effects is a balance, so that among the ten workers there were, again, three deaths from lung cancer at ages 55, 60, and 65, but in different men. What is the effect of workplace exposure?

Clearly the measurable effect would be nil, unless it were possible to distinguish between those cases saved from a smoking-attributable death and those cases caused by the carcinogen. All of the exposed lung cancer deaths are attributable in a mechanistic sense to the occupational exposure. Three deaths were also prevented, so that the magnitude of the disease burden in the population is unchanged. Any epidemiologic measure of the relation of disease to exposure describes a net change in the population, and does not capture the effect of exposure on an individual level. No one can say on the basis of population data what fraction of exposed cases would have had their disease in the absence of exposure, nor what fraction of potential cases were averted by exposure.

The lack of a basis for individual causal inference is not limited to situations where the overall effect is absent, nor is it simply a matter of substitution of cases. As an alternative to the example above, imagine that three exposed men died of lung cancer at ages 50, 55, and 60. If the effect of exposure had been to change the age at death from 65 to 50 years in a single man, we might be tempted to say that a third of the lung cancer mortality had been affected by exposure. If the effect had been to shift each death forward by five years, then the timing of all the deaths would be attributable to

---

22. The example is reworked from Robins JM and Greenland S, Estimability and estimation of excess and etiologic fractions. Statist Med 1989; in press. See also Greenland S and Robins JM, Conceptual problems in the definition and interpretation of attributable fractions. Am J Epidemiol 1988;128:1185-97

exposure. The two situations, though quite different from the perspective of the men involved, are epidemiologically indistinguishable.

What then of the tenets with which the chapter opened? If epidemiology is to make any contribution to science, then generalizability and the reciprocal relation between individual and group phenomena must hold. There is no guarantee that they do hold, and so they must be tested, through replication of studies. If differences in disease frequency are the result of general processes that have been adequately tagged by the comparisons undertaken, then similar comparisons elsewhere should yield similar results. The modulations of exposure effect outlined above result from the superimposed effects of characteristics or exposures that bear only a coincidental relation to the exposure under study. In the first example, the apparent effect of workplace exposure would be very different in smoking and nonsmoking men. In the second, the apparent effect would be sensitive to the baseline disease rates and to the time periods at which men are observed in both scenarios.

When the measure of comparison, be it a difference or a ratio or one drawn from a statistical model, does not correspond to some essential feature of the disease generating process, then it is unlikely that the results of the same comparison undertaken in different populations will be the same. Neither ratio nor difference measures capture the acceleration of disease posed in the second example given above, and the epidemiologist will find it difficult to reproduce the "effect" under circumstances that vary only slightly in the timing of observation. Replication of results in different populations is not proof that a studied relation is valid, since it is possible to repeat mistakes. Nonetheless, replicability is a strong test of the hypothesis of generalizability, and relations that withstand the test are better substantiated than those that have not been subjected to it.

# 3

# Study Types

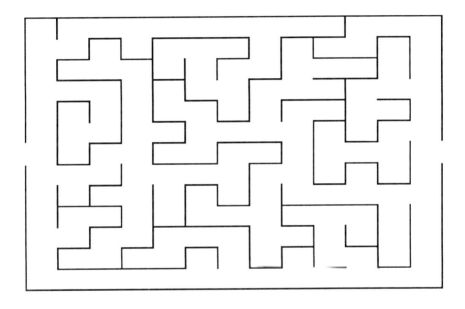

Investigators who want to learn about disease prevalence or incidence content themselves with observations made on small portions of the populations that they would like to characterize. The process of choosing study subjects from the populations of interest is known as *sampling*. The strategies used to carry out sampling define three classes of epidemiologic study: the *survey*, the *cohort study*, and the *case-control study*. Each is valid, has its own logic, has its pitfalls. The purpose of the present chapter is to introduce the three study types, with an emphasis on their interrelations. Chapters 4 and 5 will explore cohort and case-control studies in greater detail.

## Surveys

Surveys describe prevalence. The sampling that yields survey data has the goal of obtaining a study population that is a replica in miniature of a *source population*[23] (Figure 3.1).

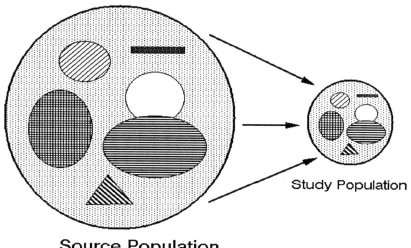

## Source Population

**Figure 3.1** A survey

**Source population.** *The individuals about whose experience or condition a study yields data are the source population. A source population is defined by the identity of the individuals whom it comprises and by the time periods during which each individual is considered to be a member.*

**Study population.** *The study population is the group of individuals that an investigator observes.*

**Sampling.** *The process of selecting a study population from a source population, with the goal of learning about characteristics of the source population, is known as sampling.*

---

23. The source population is also sometimes called the "base population," a term that connotes the role of the source population as the base upon which the structure of a study is erected.

Surveys generally address themselves to the status of individuals, assessed at a single point in time. In surveys, measurements that might be too expensive to make on the entire source population can be made in a study population, and knowledge of the sampling scheme allows you to generalize the particular data obtained to the larger group.

**Table 3.1** Prevalence of blood pressure readings among white males aged 35-44 years in the United States in 1970 (percent)

| Systolic blood pressure | Diastolic blood pressure (mm Hg) | | | | | |
|---|---|---|---|---|---|---|
| | Under 70 | 70- | 80- | 90- | 100- | Over 109 |
| Under 110 | 2.3 | 4.7 | 1.7 | - | - | - |
| 110-119 | 1.5 | 6.9 | 9.1 | 0.6 | - | - |
| 120-129 | 0.4 | 6.1 | 14.9 | 5.2 | 0.1 | - |
| 130-139 | 0.4 | 3.8 | 10.5 | 7.0 | 2.6 | 0.3 |
| 140-149 | 0.2 | 0.1 | 3.4 | 4.4 | 2.9 | 0.9 |
| 150-159 | - | - | 0.4 | 2.5 | 2.4 | 0.8 |
| 160-169 | - | - | 0.2 | 0.6 | 0.1 | 1.4 |
| 170 and over | - | 0.5 | - | - | 0.2 | 0.8 |

Table 3.1 is drawn from a National Center for Health Statistics survey. While it purports to describe all white males aged 35-44 years in the United States in 1970, the measurements pertain only to some thousand men, chosen as the study population from a source population that included all white males in the United States. The entries in the table are the percentages of the full sample found in each category of systolic and diastolic blood pressure.

Prevalence data are key to health planning, and they provide the underpinnings for the standards on which most diagnostic practice rests. However useful, prevalence tends to be dissatisfying to someone who is looking into the origins of disease, because it offers little insight into the direction of causal relations. The result is seldom persuasive, in part because of concern about differential mortality rates.[24] Figure 3.2[25] presents an example of cross-sectional data that tantalize because they fall just short.

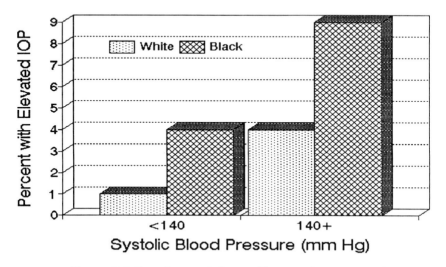

Systolic Blood Pressure (mm Hg)

**Figure 3.2** Prevalence of elevated intraocular pressure ($\geq$22 mm Hg) according to race and systolic hypertension (females)

Elevated intraocular pressure is more common in hypertensives and in blacks. Does systolic hypertension lead to (or at least predate) ocular hypertension? Are there common factors giving rise to both? Do white and black women differ in their reasons for developing an elevated IOP? The data are silent: they give an end result, not the natural history.

### Closed Cohort Studies

It is the search for cause and effect that leads to the introduction of elapsed time into epidemiologic studies. The most direct form of this introduction is in the cohort study, whose most classical form is the *closed cohort*, the nonrandomized cousin of a clinical trial.

---

24. See the discussion of survivor cohorts in Chapter 4.

25. Klein BE, Klein R. Intraocular pressure and cardiovascular risk variables. Arch Ophthalmol 1981;99:837-9

**Cohort.** *Any group of individuals whose disease or mortality is measured over time is a cohort.*

**Closed cohort.** *A closed cohort consists of individuals who are followed from a defined starting point to a defined end point. The membership of the group does not change, apart from mortality, from the beginning of observation to the end.*[26]

The term "cohort" was originally a Roman military term: a cohort was one-tenth of a legion. Typically the members of a cohort would be recruited from young men of a single age from one locale. The cohort would then undergo attrition, never being replenished, and would be disbanded when the term of enlistment was over. The word "cohort" has come to be used in epidemiology to designate individuals whose experience we observe in order to learn about the occurrence of disease.

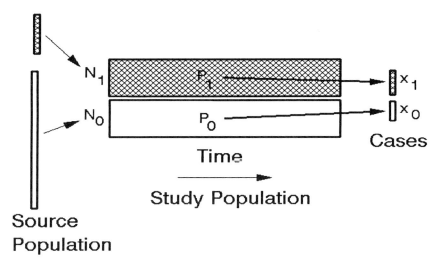

**Figure 3.3** A closed cohort study

Typically, closed cohort studies begin with study groups of approximately equal size, one of which has undergone some exposure or experience that is thought to influence the risk of acquiring disease. The study groups "1" and "0" in Figure 3.3 are followed through time,

---

26. Closed cohorts are also referred to as "fixed" cohorts.

and eventually cases of disease ($x_1$ and $x_0$) begin to appear. Notice from Figure 3.3 that the sizes of the exposed and unexposed study groups ($N_1$ and $N_0$ respectively) are not necessarily at all representative of the relative numbers of exposed and unexposed people in the source population. Nor is the person time of experience ($P_1$ and $P_0$) in the two populations "representative" of any particular distribution of person time elsewhere. Through subject selection there is an intentional distortion of the exposure distribution in the study population relative to the source population. The distortion serves to increase the efficiency of the study by reducing the imbalance in expenditures for the observation of exposed and unexposed subjects.

**Table 3.3** Available comparisons in closed cohort studies

|  | Difference | Ratio |
| --- | --- | --- |
| Cumulative incidence | $\dfrac{x_1}{N_1} - \dfrac{x_0}{N_0}$ | $\dfrac{x_1}{N_1} / \dfrac{x_0}{N_0}$ |
| Incidence rate | $\dfrac{x_1}{P_1} - \dfrac{x_0}{P_0}$ | $\dfrac{x_1}{P_1} / \dfrac{x_0}{P_0}$ |

At the end of follow-up, the occurrence of disease can be measured and compared as shown in Table 3.3. Cumulative incidences are the proportions of persons in the original cohorts who become diseased. Incidence rates are the numbers of cases per unit of person time (e.g. person years) at risk. Cumulative incidences are the closed cohort measures that are easiest to interpret: they answer a question that is implicit in the structure of the study: what proportion becomes ill? Most of us see our own futures as tiny closed cohorts, with risk interpreted in a probabilistic sense.

In order for any statement of risk to be interpretable, it must be presented with a specification of the elapsed time over which the cumulative incidence is manifest. The "risk of relapse" or the "risk of myocardial infarction" are meaningless by themselves: they need to be fleshed out to the "risk of relapse within the first year following successful induction of a disease remission" or the "risk of having an MI between the ages of 50 and 59."

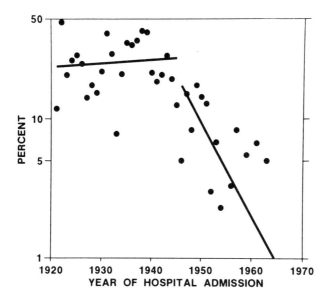

**Figure 3.4** Five-year case-fatality rates for patients less than 15 years of age with rheumatic carditis

**Example 3.1.** *Case-fatality for rheumatic carditis.*[27]

Patients with rheumatic heart disease who were admitted to the House of the Good Samaritan in Boston at age 15 years or younger were followed in order to determine the course of their disease. Two outcomes were assessed at the end of five years' follow-up: death and clinical resolution of all murmurs. There were 2090 patients, of whom 339 died in the five years following first admission. Figure 3.4 displays the five year *case fatality rates* (i.e. cumulative incidences of death over five years) for each closed cohort defined by hospital admission in each calendar year from 1921 through 1970. The black dots represent the observed cohort-specific case fatality rates,[28] and the dark lines are

27. Massell BF, Chute CG, Walker AM, Kurland GS. Penicillin and the marked decrease in morbidity and mortality from rheumatic fever in the United States. N Engl J Med 1988;318:280-6

28. There were no deaths after 1963, so that the location of the dots for later years is outside the range graphed in Figure 3.3.

estimates of the linear components of the secular trends. There is an evident inflection in the trend around the years 1945 and 1946. Figure 3.5 shows the proportion of loss of all cardiac murmurs (i.e. clinical recovery) over the same periods in the same cohorts. There were 343 such children. Again, there is a discontinuity just after the end of the second World War. The cumulative incidence difference, comparing 1945 with 1946, was estimated at 13 percent. In all likelihood, the source of the abrupt changes in Figures 3.4 and 3.5 was the widespread civilian availability of penicillin. Trends in national mortality rates from rheumatic fever showed the same discontinuity, with an acceleration in the rate of decline after 1946.

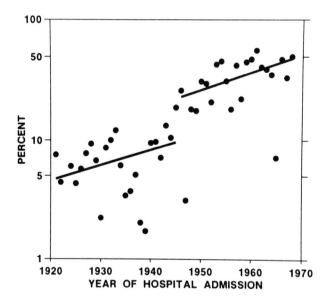

**Figure 3.5** Proportion of rheumatic carditis patients less than 15 years of age in whom all evidence of murmurs disappeared within five years

The foregoing example describes cumulative incidences. As indicated in Chapter 1, for closed cohort studies, (and for clinical trials), the incidence rate of disease can be calculated simply as the proportion becoming diseased, divided by the average time of disease-free follow-up. For closed cohort studies, rate calculations may appear to provide an unnecessary flourish, but there is an important class of cohort studies in which incidence rates are the only measure that is directly accessible: these are *open cohort studies.*

### Open Cohort Studies

Consider a study of smoking in men aged 50-59. For five calendar years, we recruit both smokers and nonsmokers into the study. We follow them during the same period: smokers and non-smokers in the appropriate age range are observed for the occurrence of myocardial infarction for as long as they remain eligible. This study situation differs in crucial respects from the closed cohort design:

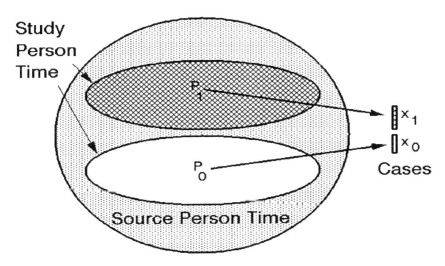

**Figure 3.6** An open cohort study

(1) "Exposure" does not represent an event, fixed in time, but rather a status, which continues over time, of being a smoker or

a nonsmoker.[29]

(2) There is no fixed ending time for observation.

(3) Subjects can enter the study at any time, and they may leave it (by dying or leaving town or through termination of the study) at any time.

**Open cohort.** *An open cohort is a cohort whose studied composition may change with the passage of time.*[30]

Even in a closed cohort, the composition of the population may change with time prior to the end of follow-up, due to the onset of disease or to change in the defining exposure. The difference between an open and a closed cohort is that in an open cohort the evolving population composition (describable in terms of persons and exposures) is directly monitored and becomes the studied experience. Allowance for change in the observed population opens up the possibility of cohort studies that can be adapted to populations that do not fit the static presumptions of closed cohort analysis.

In an open cohort, cases arise out of a pool of human experience whose size is measured in units of person time. The $x_1$ and $x_0$ of Figure 3.6 represent the cases that arise out of the $P_1$ exposed and $P_0$ unexposed person years contributed by exposed and unexposed persons to the study person-time. The study person-time in turn may represent just a portion of the source person-time, that is, the person-time experience of the source population.

Although open cohort studies permit more flexible designs, they do not offer all the comparisons that can be derived from closed cohorts. The three conditions outlined above render cumulative incidence differences or ratios unavailable as measures of disease frequency: you cannot talk about "MIs per 100 men" when a man may represent a quantity of observation that ranges anywhere from days to years. You can, however, still talk about incidence rates, as

---

29. It would be possible to perform a closed cohort study of smokers and nonsmokers. The chief advantage of closed cohort designs is that they permit a direct and natural estimation of risk (c.f. Table 3.3). For the closed cohort design to offer an advantage in this example, there should be the achievement of some state, such as "smoker" or "smoker for 20 years" as the definition of $t_0$. The risk over a specified interval following such a well defined $t_0$ could be a generally useful figure; the risk over the same interval following an otherwise unrestricted study entry date is unlikely to be of general interest.

30. The term "dynamic cohort" is sometimes used to describe open cohorts.

**Table 3.4** Available comparisons in open cohort studies

|  | Difference | Ratio |
|---|---|---|
| Cumulative incidence | * | * |
| Incidence rate | $\dfrac{x_1}{P_1} - \dfrac{x_0}{P_0}$ | $\dfrac{x_1}{P_1} \Big/ \dfrac{x_0}{P_0}$ |

\* Not defined for open cohort studies

"MIs per man year (or man month or 100 man years) of observation."
The available comparisons between groups are reduced to those in
Table 3.4.

**Example 3.2.**  *Vasectomy and myocardial infarction.*[31]

Table 3.5 presents the results of an open cohort study of the
incidence of myocardial infarction in vasectomized men.  Men
in an HMO who had undergone vasectomy between 1963 and
1978 were observed while they were members of the HMO for
the occurrence of myocardial infarction.  Their experience was
compared to that of a group of HMO members without vasectomy.
Men with and without vasectomies could move between age
categories so that each could contribute person years of experience to several age categories.

This open cohort study is based on a well-defined list of persons,
and could readily incorporate a clear $t_0$, the date of vasectomy.  What
makes this an open cohort is the opportunity for men to enter or
leave follow-up at any moment.  The opportunity to change some
aspect of their "exposure" (in this case age) with every moment would
also be sufficient to define this as an open cohort.  The incidence
rate analysis is characteristic of an open cohort study, but it does
not define it, since closed cohort experience can also be subjected
to incidence rate analysis.

31. Walker AM, Jick H, Hunter JR, McEvoy J.  Vasectomy and nonfatal myocardial
infarction: Continued observation indicates no elevation of risk.  J Urol 1983;130:936-8

**Table 3.5** First time myocardial infarction rates in vasectomized and nonvasectomized men

| Age | Cases | Person Years | Rate per 1,000 |
|---|---|---|---|
| *Vasectomized* | | | |
| 35-44 | 14 | 16,806 | 0.8 |
| 45-54 | 24 | 8,133 | 3.0 |
| 55-64 | 7 | 1,700 | 4.1 |
| Total | 45 | 26,639 | 1.7 |
| *Not Vasectomized* | | | |
| 35-44 | 56 | 83,057 | 0.7 |
| 45-54 | 110 | 40,971 | 2.7 |
| 55-64 | 49 | 8,570 | 5.7 |
| Total | 215 | 132,598 | 1.6 |

Cohort studies provide an opportunity for direct observation of time relations and are well-adapted to the study of relatively common disease outcomes. However, observation for even moderately rare diseases that do not occur within a short time requires large numbers of subjects (numbering in the thousands or ten of thousands) observed over many years. When the occurrence of disease is not a common event, the expense of maintaining information on a large enough cohort of persons at risk may be prohibitive. Investigators deal with this common situation through a study design whose cardinal feature is that data are not collected on all persons, but rather on samples of the diseased and nondiseased populations.

## Case-Control Studies

Figure 3.7 presents a schematic picture of the relation of a case-control study to an underlying open cohort. Illustrated is the common situation in which the sampling fraction for cases is 100 percent. As before, there is experience among persons exposed and among those unexposed. As before, cases arise out of the pool of experience: $x_1$ exposed and $x_0$ unexposed. If $P_1$ and $P_0$ were known, the ratio of rates in exposed versus unexposed person time could be calculated as $(x_1/P_1)/(x_0/P_0)$, which equals algebraically $(x_1/x_0)/(P_1/P_0)$. $(x_1/x_0)$ is called the exposure odds among the cases; $(P_1/P_0)$ is the exposure odds in the source population.

**Exposure odds.** *The number of exposed persons divided by the number of unexposed persons in a group yields the exposure odds. The exposure odds in a pool of person time are obtained by dividing the amount of exposed person-time by the amount of unexposed person-time.*

In both open cohort studies and case-control studies, the exposure odds in cases is observed directly. The difference between an open cohort study and the corresponding case-control study is that the exposure odds in the source population $(P_1/P_0)$ are not observed in the latter design. Instead, in the case-control study, the exposure odds in the source population are estimated from a sample of person days. Like a marine biologist counting different species of algae, we dip a test tube into the pool of experience of an open cohort to learn its composition. In so doing, we return to the cross-sectional survey discussed at the beginning of the chapter. The goal is to sample a small proportion of the population giving rise to the cases in such a way as to estimate the exposure odds in that source population.

Note that since we are sampling person time, the sampled population is a population of person days, defined operationally as specified days in the lives of specified individuals. Both the person and the date are chosen by some suitably random procedure. The sampled group of person days is called the control series. The persons whose days are sampled are called the *controls*.

**Controls.** *The controls in a case-control study are a group of persons whose exposure status collectively provides information about the distribution of exposure in the persons or person time giving rise to the cases.*

Table 3.6 gives the layout of data from a case-control study. The ratio of exposed to unexposed controls $(y_1/y_0)$ is an estimate of $(P_1/P_0)$. The incidence rate ratio from a case-control study is derived then as

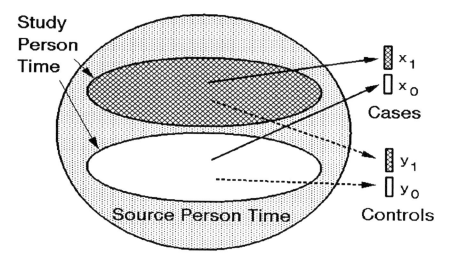

**Figure 3.7** A case-control study that arises from an open cohort

$$RR = \frac{IR_1}{IR_0} = \frac{x_1/P_1}{x_0/P_0}$$

$$\doteq \frac{x_1 y_0}{x_0 y_1}$$

The symbol "$\doteq$" means "approximately equal to." The approximation involved has to do with the additional, statistical error that results from taking a sample of all person days to represent the total. The quantity in the last line is the ratio of exposure odds in cases to the exposure odds in controls, and is referred to as the *odds ratio* (*OR*). The odds ratio in a case-control study is an estimate of the rate ratio in the source population giving rise to cases and controls.

Case-control studies are also conducted in situations for which the most natural corresponding cohort study is the closed cohort. In perinatal epidemiology, an infant's health status might typically be assessed at 30 days of life. If cases were drawn from those who had died, then controls would be chosen at random from those who have survived. When the controls are drawn from the healthy survivors of a closed cohort and when the cases are a small proportion of the

**Table 3.6** Data layout for a case-control study

|          | Exposed | Unexposed |
|----------|:-------:|:---------:|
| Cases    | $x_1$   | $x_0$     |
| Controls | $y_1$   | $y_0$     |

$$RR \doteq OR = \frac{x_1 y_0}{x_0 y_1}$$

total study subjects, the ratio $y_1/y_0$ provides an estimate of the ratio of exposed to unexposed persons in the source population ($N_1/N_0$), so that the cumulative incidence ratio can be estimated as

$$CIR = \frac{CI_1}{CI_0} = \frac{x_1/N_1}{x_0/N_0}$$

$$\doteq \frac{x_1 y_0}{x_0 y_1}$$

The approximation indicated on the last line refers both to the statistical uncertainty and to the approximation taken from the use of exposure odds in the controls as an estimate of the exposure odds in the source population. The numbers of exposed and unexposed persons in the control series are used to estimate the ratio of exposed to unexposed persons in the source population.

Notice that the moment as of which the exposure status of the controls is assessed depends on whether they are drawn from an underlying cohort that is open or one that is closed. In the latter, the exposure status of interest is that which characterizes each control as of $t_0$, the initial time defining cohort eligibility. When the controls are drawn from open cohorts, the exposure status of each control is relevant only on the day(s) sampled when the controls are drawn from an open cohort.

The relative measures of disease occurrence derivable from a case-control study are displayed in Table 3.7.

**Table 3.7** Available comparisons in case-control studies

|  | Difference | Ratio |
|---|---|---|
| Cumulative incidence | * | $\dfrac{x_1 y_0}{x_0 y_1}$ |
| Incidence rate | * | $\dfrac{x_1 y_0}{x_0 y_1}$ |

* Not defined in case-control studies

All case-control studies can be seen as being carried out within some body of cohort experience. Often, the cohort giving rise to the cases can be ill-defined, and the consequent problems of definition of a proper control series can be difficult, even intractable if the source population for cases is sufficiently elusive. These issues will be addressed further in Chapter 6, but for the moment, note that in the past many case-control studies have been carried out in situations in which the source population was very poorly characterized. In order to distinguish their work from such high-risk adventures, investigators who conducted case-control sampling within well-defined cohorts have sometimes used the term *nested case-control studies*. Think of the sampling scheme as being nestled snugly within the structured confines of a well-monitored cohort.

**Nested** *describes a case-control study for which the source population is one whose person time (open cohort) or persons (closed cohort) has been previously identified and enumerated for research purposes.*

The term is sometimes used more loosely to characterize any case-control study carried out within a well-characterized cohort.[32]

---

32. As a minor esthetic point, it seems a pity to look for qualifying terms such as "nested" to set apart studies that are the standard of good practice. Why not reserve the descriptors for designs that fall below the mark? Alvin Feinstein's term "trohoc" ("cohort" spelled backwards) captured the spirit of designs that looked backwards from disease status, with no regard for the source population that gave rise to cases.

**Table 3.8** Perforated peptic ulcer and prior use of cimetidine or antacids

|                   | Prior use | No prior use |
| ----------------- | --------- | ------------ |
| Perforated ulcer  | 15        | 25           |
| Controls          | 30        | 250          |

$$RR \doteq \frac{(15)(250)}{(25)(30)} = 5.0$$

**Example 3.3.** *Cimetidine, antacids, and peptic ulcer.*[33]

In a case-control study of the determinants of perforated peptic ulcer among the members of the Group Health Cooperative of Puget Sound (GHC), previous use of pharmaceuticals was compared between patients suffering a perforation and other members of the health plan who had a similar age-sex distribution. The cases' drug histories were abstracted from the GHC pharmacy records up to the date of perforation, and the controls' histories were abstracted up to a date that was random and different for each control, but which fell into the period of case accrual. Table 3.8 presents the numbers of cases and controls according to their previous use of cimetidine or antacids.

The data in Table 3.8 lead to the estimate that the incidence rate of perforated peptic ulcer was five times higher in persons who used antacids or cimetidine than in those who did not. The association in all probability does not reflect a dangerous side effect of the drugs under study. Rather both are markers of the presence of earlier peptic ulcer disease, which is a very strong predictor of perforated ulcer.

**Directionality**

Frequently the terms "cohort" and "case control" are confused with "prospective" and "retrospective." The tendency is a natural one, since many of the most famous cohort studies have in fact been prospective. The Framingham Heart Study is a notable example, in

33. Jick SS, Perera DR, Walker AM, Jick H. Non-steroidal anti-inflammatory drugs and hospital admission for perforated peptic ulcer. Lancet 1987;ii:380-2

which early middle-aged adults were identified in the early 1950s, and have been observed ever since. Most important case-control studies, beginning with the earliest investigations of smoking and lung cancer, have been retrospective. Nonetheless these terms, which describe the relation in time between the researcher and the object of study are quite independent of the sampling design.

**Prospective.** *A prospective study is one in which the disease events under study occur after the protocol for data collection has been implemented.*

**Retrospective.** *A retrospective study is one in which the protocol is implemented after the disease events have occurred.*

Cohort studies are frequently retrospective. The groups to be compared are defined by exposures that occurred in the distant past, and data on subsequent health events is drawn from vital statistics or medical records extending up to the date of data collection. This is typical for occupational cohort studies, and is becoming more common in other areas as long-term medical records become available for special population groups. The vasectomy study of Table 3.5 was a retrospective cohort study carried out inside a health maintenance organization.[34] More important than the time orientation of a study is the quality of the data that it yields. The greatest potential advantage of a prospective study is that the investigator can arrange the administration and data collection so that the necessary information flows into the study in a usable form. A prospective study in which the data flow is incomplete or poorly monitored has no advantage over a retrospective study carried out in an "information rich" environment.

---

34. Often studies are designed with both retrospective and prospective collection of data. A useful neologism to designate such designs is "ambispective."

# 4

# Time

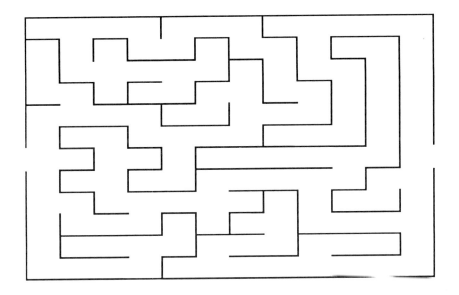

Of all the characteristics of experience that are recorded in epidemiologic studies, those related to time are measured with the greatest accuracy. Functions of time serve as markers of biological processes and can be used as surrogates for nonbiological phenomena. The purpose of this chapter is to review ways in which time can be interpreted in observational research. The first major role for time is in the classification of exposures and their effects on humans. Here time may stand in for cumulative exposure, for latency or induction periods, or for the intensity of an exposure that has changed with calendar period. Similarly time may classify persons, by defining susceptibility or concomitant determinants of risk. Time finally may characterize our ability to observe or record events that are the objects of study.

**Table 4.1** Pneumoconiosis among crocidolite miners in Western Australia

| Employment duration | Heavy exposure | | | Medium exposure | | |
|---|---|---|---|---|---|---|
| | N | x | % | N | x | % |
| <6 months | 2000 | 12 | 0.6 | 1750 | 7 | 0.4 |
| 6mo - <1yr | 529 | 9 | 1.7 | 330 | 1 | 0.3 |
| 1yr - <2yr | 338 | 23 | 6.8 | 250 | 1 | 0.4 |
| 2yr - <3yr | 141 | 23 | 16.3 | 109 | 5 | 4.6 |
| 3yr - <4yr | 74 | 18 | 24.3 | 43 | 3 | 7.0 |
| 4yr - <5yr | 84 | 33 | 39.3 | 47 | 5 | 10.6 |
| ≥5 years | 55 | 36 | 65.4 | 40 | 16 | 40.0 |

N - Number observed    x - Number with pneumoconiosis    % = 100x/N

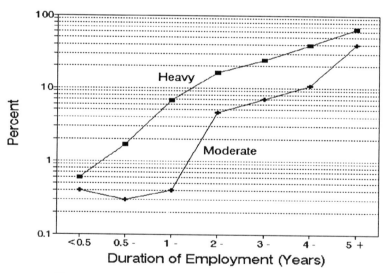

**Figure 4.1** Prevalence of pneumoconiosis among crocidolite miners in Western Australia. Data from Table 4.1.

## Time Characterizes Exposure and Exposure Effects

When exposure to an agent that may cause disease is continuous or nearly so over stretch of time, then the duration of exposure can stand as a proxy for the accumulated exposure dose. The situation arises commonly with occupational and environmental toxins, but can apply equally well to medicines taken regularly, or indeed to any personal habit, such as smoking or alcohol consumption, that may vary little over a period of time.

**Cumulative exposure.** *The cumulative exposure from time $t_0$ to time $t_1$ for an individual is the summation of all exposures endured from $t_0$ up until $t_1$.*

**Example 4.1.** *Pneumoconiosis in crocidolite miners.*[35]

Hobbs et al. studied the prevalence of pneumoconiosis in former crocidolite miners in Western Australia. Using company and pension records they identified a cohort of 7000 men ever employed (1938-1966), with dates of employment and jobs held. The eventual appearance of disease was identified from pneumoconiosis boards (which were required to certify cases for compensation), cancer registries, master patient indices of hospitals, hospital morbidity abstracts, and death records. Workers were classed according to their total duration of employment in the mines, the typical intensity of their exposure to crocidolite dust, and their final disease status, as shown in Table 4.1 and Figure 4.1.

In effect this was a study of the risk of pneumoconiosis through a time that was considered to represent the exhaustion of the effects of mining.[36] Since there were only the coarsest data available on exposure intensity, the most accurate summary of total numbers of respired asbestos fibers is given by the duration of work. For crocidolite, cumulative exposure has a particular biologic appeal. Inhaled fibers, once lodged in the lung, appear to remain there in perpetuity. The same is true of amosite asbestos, but not of chrysotile.

---

35. Hobbs MST, Woodward SD, Murphy B, Musk AW, Elder JE. The incidence of pneumoconiosis , mesothelioma and other respiratory cancer in men engaged in mining and milling crocidolite in Western Australia. In Wagner JC (ed) Biological Effects of Mineral Fibres. IARC, Lyon, 1980, pp 615-25

36. If pneumoconiosis were an infectious process and crocidolite an infectious agent, the term "attack rate" would fit perfectly here. See Chapter 5.

For both heavy and medium exposure, risk appears to have increased with duration of exposure. There is also some hint of a threshold: at less than two years' exposure to the medium level jobs there appears to have been no increase in risk, while the same periods presented a tenfold increase among the heavily exposed.

If exposure does vary with time, and if the period-specific levels of exposure can be ascertained, then summed times of exposure, weighted by relative exposure intensity, still provide a measure of cumulative exposure. The use of relative exposure measures is often found in the retrospective cohort studies common in occupational health research. Exposures to possible workplace toxins may have occurred years before quantitative measurements were feasible, but historical documents and the recollections of workers may nonetheless be sufficient to provide a rough calibration of relative intensity. Example 4.3, which appears later on, incorporates observation times weighted by estimated relative exposures to derive a semiquantitative cumulative exposure.

Closed cohort studies such as that of Hobbs, above, typically encompass a follow-up time during which all the effects of exposure are expected to play themselves out. Open cohort studies, by contrast, often permit the observation of blocks of person-time that accrue before the effects of past exposure become manifest. These intervals of no evident disease comprise the time during which pathogenic mechanisms set in motion by the exposure are working toward the production of manifest disease, and the time during which disease, though present, is not yet manifest. The former interval is the *induction period*; the portion of the induction period during which disease is present but unmanifest is the time of *latency*. Both induction period and latency are properly applied only to persons destined eventually to become diseased. As a practical matter, they therefore describe only the history of persons who have become diseased.

**Induction period.** *The induction period is the time required for the effects of a specific exposure to become manifest.*

**Table 4.2** Mortality from mesothelioma in Canadian asbestos-cement factory workers

| Time since first exposure | Man years P | Mesothelioma x | Mortality R |
|---|---|---|---|
| 15 - 19 years | 1182 | 1 | 0.8 |
| 20 - 24 years | 1061 | 4 | 3.7 |
| 25 - 29 years | 555 | 5 | 9.0 |
| 30 - 34 years | 104 | 1 | 9.6 |

P - Man years at risk   x - Mesothelioma deaths   R - Deaths per 1000 man years at risk

**Example 4.2.** *Mesothelioma among asbestos cement factory workers.*[37]

Finkelstein traced the mortality of Canadian asbestos-cement factory workers. The cohort was assembled from company files, and was confirmed as complete by cross-checking union seniority lists and radiographic surveillance lists. The cohort was restricted to men with at least one year employment who were hired before 1960 and who had passed at least 15 years since their date of hire. Vital status was obtained from the Canadian Mortality Data Base, from driver's license records, and from the U.S. Immigration and Naturalization Service. Each worker's contribution to the person time under observation was categorized according to time since first hire. The incidence of mesothelioma rose rapidly through the period from 15 to 29 years after first exposure, and then leveled off (Table 4.2).

The induction periods for the 11 cases of mesothelioma cannot be ascertained exactly from Table 4.2, which presents the data only in intervals. Approximately, the induction periods ranged from 15 to 34 years. Note that there is no single induction period that characterizes mesothelioma in asbestos cement workers; there is rather a collection of intervals, whose relative frequency will be determined both by the pathophysiology of human response to the exposure and by the durations of follow-up of the men in the cohort.

37. Finkelstein MM. Mortality among long-term employees of an Ontario asbestos-cement factory. Br J Ind Med 1983;40:138-44

Finkelstein's work is an example of an open cohort study. Workers contributed person time of follow-up to each of the interval categories of Table 4.2 for so long as they were under observation in each category. The persons contributing time to successive categories of time since first exposure were largely the same individuals.[38] Contrast this to Table 4.1, in which the categories of exposure were mutually exclusive insofar as individuals are concerned. In Table 4.2 the mutual exclusivity pertains to the classification of person time.

The interval from first exposure to time of observation is often called *latency* in the literature of occupational epidemiology; the "latency" of disease onset is the term used to denote the induction period. "Latency" in its ordinary English usage implies that disease is present but unobserved. The implication is at odds with the technical meaning in occupational studies during most of the interval between first exposure and onset for diseased persons, and during all of the time of observation for persons who never develop disease. Since the ordinary usage is a valuable and reasonably precise method of denoting a disease state with no observable manifestations, "latency" should be used in its common sense in epidemiology as well. However, because there is an entrenched history of the nonintuitive usage in studies of occupational health, authors and readers should be clear which meaning of latency is intended.

**Latent.** *A disease that is present but not symptomatic is latent.*[39]

**Latency.** *The time interval during which a disease is latent. Also, in occupational epidemiology, the interval from first exposure to observation.*

When an induction period is present, incidence rates rise only after a time lag following the onset of exposure. This phenomen of delayed manifestation of causally attributable events is sometimes called the *residual effect* of an exposure.

**Residual effect.** *The subsequent changes in disease incidence that are attributable to an exposure are said to be the residual effect of that exposure.*

---

38. See Tables 3.5, 4.5, and 5.2 for other examples of this characteristic property of open cohorts: the divisibility of persons.

39. The theory of screening tests employs a related concept, the "detectable preclinical phase" of disease. Whether or not a latent disease is in its detectable preclinical phase depends on the available means of detection.

Cumulative exposure, induction period, and residual effect all derive from a central concept of the influence of exposure on disease occurrence. Imagine each increment of time as characterized by an isolated element of exposure whose effect on incidence is cast into the future, typically as a function that rises, plateaus, and then falls. Let the effect of each one of these exposure increments be super-imposed on the effects of all other exposure increments in a simple additive way. The hazard[40] at any moment is then the sum of the hazards attributable to all past exposures. If the hazard function attributable to a particular past exposure quantum has fallen to zero at a given moment, then the particular past exposure is without residual effect.

Cumulative exposure is a linear predictor of hazard for as long as the residual effects of past exposures are not changing with the passage of time and can be summed onto one another. During such a period the hazard will rise in direct proportion to the total prior exposure. The minimum induction period is not a well-defined interval, but corresponds rather to the time elapsed until the summed residual effects from all prior exposures become high enough to result in observable disease. The residual effect of the cumulative exposure and the observed induction periods are the playing out of the summed residual effects of past exposures over the duration of follow-up.

**Example 4.3.** *Colon cancer and the production of acrylic sheet.*[41]

Jobs in a factory engaged in the production of acrylic sheet prior to 1945 were classified according to the estimated vapor phase exposure to acrylate monomers. Exposure was scored on a scale running from 1 to 5, and was based on the recollections, some 40 years later, of workers who had been familiar with the plant. Exposure essentially ceased after 1945 because of changes in the manufacturing process. Cumulative exposure to acrylate monomers up to any point in time was calculated for each man by multiplying the exposure score in each of his jobs by the duration of that job, and summing the result over all jobs up to the time in question. The highest cumulative exposure was 20

---

40. The hazard is the expected value of the incidence rate; it is the unobservable parameter of which the observed incidence rate provides an estimate. See Chapter 7 for more on hazard and on the relation between parameters and estimates.

41. Walker AM, Cohen A, Loughlin J, DeFonso L, Rothman KR. Mortality from cancers of the colon and rectum in workers exposed to ethylacrylate and methylmethacrylate. Scand J Work Environ Hlth 1991;

**Table 4.3**  Deaths from colon cancer in relation to the time since accumulation of 15 units of exposure to acrylates

|  | Not exposed to acrylates | Exposed to less than 15 units | Years since achieving 15 units of exposure | | |
|---|---|---|---|---|---|
|  |  |  | <5 | 5-14 | 15+ |
| Incidence[1] | 40 | 62 | 0 | 11 | 89 |
| Deaths observed | 11 | 26 | 0 | 1 | 11 |
| Deaths expected[2] | 11.48 | 19.81 | 0.11 | 0.88 | 4.58 |
| Ratio obs/exp | 0.96 | 1.3 | 0 | 1.1 | 2.4 |
| Person years | 23,487 | 51,552 | 1,812 | 5,040 | 5,531 |

[1] Deaths per 100,000 person years among men aged 30-84 years, standardized to the age distribution of person time in the full cohort

[2] Expectations were calculated on the basis of contemporaneous local mortality rates for cancer of the colon.

units. All men who achieved 15 units of exposure did so by working three or more years in a single high-exposure aspect of production, the "boil out" process. Men who had worked in the plant for at least 10 months were traced, and deaths from colon cancer were identified from a variety of sources. For the results presented in Table 4.3, person time was accumulated in categories defined by age, calendar year, and the time since achievement of a cumulative exposure of at least 15 units. Because colon cancer was not expected to (and did not) lead to any deaths under the age of 30 years, and because there was essentially no experience to summarize from the age of 85 years on, the data in Table 4.3 concern only person years from age 30 to 84.

The partitioning of person time in Table 4.3 was chosen so as to examine the possible existence of an induction period for colon cancer following a cumulative exposure of 15 units. The data indicate that the age-standardized colon cancer rates did rise with the passage of time since the accumulation of 15 units of exposure. If the association is causal, then in Table 4.3 there is evidence for the existence of a residual effect of acrylates on colon cancer mortality, with induction periods from the completion of 15 units of exposure to death typically exceeding 15 years.

## Historical Intensity of Exposure

In most retrospective cohort studies (and essentially all case-control studies), there is a tight relation between "time since first exposure" and "era of first exposure." It is very often the case that the nature and intensity of exposure has changed in poorly documented ways with the evolution of time. Finkelstein (Example 4.2), for example, assigned the following asbestos fiber exposures to mixing operators:

| 1949 | 40.0 f/ml |
| 1969 | 20.0 f/ml |
| 1979 | 0.2 f/ml |

The meaning of the term "mixing operator" changed with the passage of time. As a result, any portrayal of the rate of asbestos-related disease in mixing operators at a fixed time, say 1985, could give the appearance of a dependence of disease on time since entry into the field, and on age, that was entirely an artifact of variations in asbestos exposure history. Proper analysis of the effect of age or time since entry into the trade would have to be done within blocks of human experience defined by exposure intensity, that is to say, defined by calendar period of entry into the trade. Necessarily such studies would have to be carried out over an extended period.

The change in the meaning of exposure with the passage of time is the origin of a *cohort effect* among the exposed. In the analysis of vital statistics data, cohort effects are variations in disease incidence, seen at all ages, that are characteristic of persons born in a particular era. The characteristics that drive cohort effects are usually in place in childhood or young adult life, but in any case, prior to the regular onset of disease occurrence in the population.

**Cohort effect.** *Changes in disease frequency that are shared by all members of a group who entered follow-up at common time constitute a cohort effect.*

Cohort effects are typically produce by shared characteristics of subgroups of the the persons under observaton.

## Changes in Cohort Composition

The deceleration in the rise of mesothelioma mortality recorded in Table 4.2 may have been due to chance. It may also have been the result of biological phenomena, such as a declining residual effect of asbestos exposure. It may also occur because the exposure categories contain different proportions of persons at high risk of death.

If the workers within each category of follow-up actually have an undocumented variety of exposure histories, and if exposure is related to continuation under follow-up for any reason, then the exposure composition of the surviving cohort change will change over time. In the present instance, particularly high levels of exposure to asbestos would lead to elevated mortality. With the passage of time, a group of workers comprising individuals with both high and low levels of exposure will selectively lose those cohort members with the higher exposures. The average intensity of exposure in the surviving portion of the cohort will be lower than that of the cohort at its inception. The change in disease patterns with time will then be that truly related to the lapse of time mixed with (that is, confounded by) changes due to the changing exposure profile of the persons who continue to be observed.

Because the cohort composition with respect to unmeasured determinants of disease does commonly evolve with the passage of time, it is useful to distinguish a cohort as it exists at some initial point of observation from one that is far removed from an initial membership-determining event.

**Inception cohort.** *The persons who are under observation at the beginning of an exposure that defines cohort membership are termed an inception cohort.*

**Survivor cohort.** *The persons who remain under observation at some point after the beginning of an exposure that defines cohort membership are a survivor cohort.*

All cohorts defined later than at birth are in some sense survivor cohorts,[42] and studies of multiple causes of disease almost necessarily identify persons who are members of survivor cohorts for some of the causes under study.

---

42. A reproductive epidemiologist might extend the definition to cohorts defined after conception.

## Susceptibility

Identical exposures may have different effects when administered to the same person at different times. The prototypical example of this phenomenon is teratogenesis.

**Example 4.4.** *Prenatal DES exposure and vaginal epithelial changes.*[43]

The DESAD (Diethylstilbesterol Adenosis) project obtained follow-up gynecologic examinations on 1340 young women identified through reviews of obstetricians' notes as having been exposed to DES (diethylstilbesterol) prenatally. At examination, the presence of macro- or microscopic changes in vaginal mucosa were noted. The project found the relation shown in Figure 4.2 between prevalence of VEC (vaginal epithelial changes) and the timing of first maternal DES exposure.

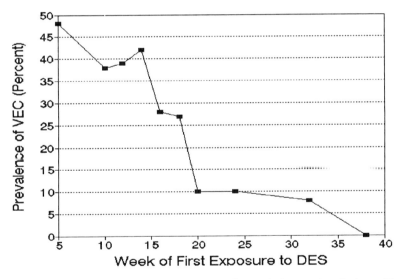

**Figure 4.2** Prevalence of VEC in relation to the timing of in utero exposure to DES

43. O'Brien PC, Noller KL, Robboy SJ, et al. Vaginal epithelial changes in young women enrolled in the National Cooperative Diethylstilbesterol Adenosis (DESAD) project. Obstet Gynecol 1979;53:300-8

It appears that exposure prior to the twentieth week of pregnancy posed a much greater risk for eventual VEC in the offspring than did exposure at a later date. The most crucial period was probably early in pregnancy, when the vaginal epithelium is being formed. The gradual diminution in risk after week 20 may represent either a decline in sensitivity of the fetal vagina to the effects of DES, or it may be an artifact of error in the ascertainment of onset of DES use, superimposed on an abrupt disappearance of susceptibility.

## Concomitant Determinants of Risk or Diagnosis

Time, measured by age, can stand as a proxy for individual characteristics that determine risk. Although many diseases occur more frequently in elderly people than in younger persons, the relation between age and incidence is entirely disease-specific, as Example 4.5 will show.

In the form of calendar year of observation, time may stand as a determinant of the risk of diagnosis among persons with a given disease status. For diseases with long induction periods, changes in the definition of disease, in the technology for diagnosing disease, or in the *a priori* expectation that a disease is present are the most important determinants of calendar-year specific changes in the risk of diagnosis.

**Example 4.5.** *Replacement estrogens and fibrocystic disease of the breast.*[44]

Jick et al examined the incidence of biopsy diagnosis of fibrocystic breast disease (FBD) in an HMO for whose members it was possible to identify use of prescription drugs. Among nonusers of replacement estrogens, they found the incidence rates graphed in Figure 4.3.

The incidence of biopsy-proven FBD declined both with age and with calendar time. The decline with age had been seen in previous studies, and may reflect a diminution in circulating estrogen levels after menopause. The decline is an example of an *age effect.*

**Age effect.** *A change in disease incidence that is due to a biological concomitant of aging is an age effect.*

44. Jick SS, Walker AM, Jick H. Conjugated estrogens and fibrocystic breast disease. Am J Epidemiol 1986;124:746-51

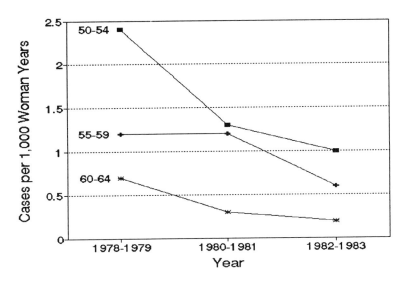

**Figure 4.3** Incidence of biopsy-proven FBD in non-users of replacement estrogens aged 50-54, 55-59, and 60-64 years

The notable in incidence of FBD decline over the six calendar years of observation in all age groups also suggests a changed definition of pathology in the female breast. Late in the 1970s, there was a campaign against what was conceived to be a misguided practice of labeling as fibrocystic "disease" a normal condition found in many women. Particularly because of the psychological burden on patients who were left with the impression that they harbored a premalignant condition, biopsies became less frequent, and a diagnosis of FBD became less frequent among biopsied women. The decline in the apparent incidence of FBD with time is an example of a *period effect*.

**Period effect.** *Changes in disease frequency that are specific to a calendar time are collectively termed a period effect.*

Period effects are most commonly the result of secular changes in the deifinition of disease or in diagnostic practice. Period effects can also result from secular changes in the prevalence of exposures that produce disease with short induction periods.

Look again at Table 4.3. A secular trend in the diagnosis of colon cancer might confound the comaprison of the incidence rates listed in the last three columns. One purpose of calculating the "Deaths expected" on the basis of calendar-year specific mortality data was to compensate for period effects.

## Diagnostic Suspicion

The proclivity to carry out a diagnostic maneuver or to make a diagnosis often varies with time in a way that is closely related to duration of exposure. For current users of replacement estrogens, Jick et al (Example 4.4) found the following crude data shown in Table 4.4.

**Table 4.4** Duration of replacement estrogen use and the incidence of fibrocystic breast disease

| Year of Use | Woman Years | FBD | Incidence |
|---|---|---|---|
| First | 1383 | 4 | 2.9 |
| Second | 1833 | 1 | 0.6 |
| Third | 1930 | 1 | 0.5 |
| Fourth | 1339 | 2 | 1.5 |
| Fifth & up | 5033 | 11 | 2.2 |

Incidence = FBD / 1000 woman years

The elevated incidence in the first year of replacement estrogen use may have resulted from increased surveillance. Women who begin use of replacement estrogens necessarily have had recent physician contact, and may be particularly willing to report breast symptoms. Replacement estrogens themselves increase breast tenderness in some women and may lead to consultation with physicians. Either mechanism can set off a chain of events that leads to a biopsy for a suspicious breast mass in a very small percentage of women. Although the motivating concern is the early detection of a possible breast cancer, the result is a final diagnosis of a benign condition (FBD) and a blip in the FBD incidence rates in the first year of replacement estrogen therapy.

The later rise in the FBD rates of Table 4.4 may also be related to an increased surveillance for possible breast cancer. In the latter part of the 1970s, there were a number of reports of an association between replacement estrogen use of long duration and breast cancer. One of those reports had been based on observations at the HMO where the FBD study was carried out. If you were a treating physician and were faced with very slightly suspicious change in the texture of the breast tissue in one of your patients, for whom would your inclination to order a biopsy be greatest? Given equal symptoms, women who were long-term users of replacement estrogens were at the highest risk for biopsy. Nonmalignant changes in lumpy breasts tended to receive the diagnosis FBD, and women who were long-term users of replacement estrogens tended to receive the diagnosis with greater frequency than others.

## Time that is Event-Free by Definition

Members of a survivor cohort have accumulated experience prior to the time at which the formal period of their observation begins. Similarly, any cohort whose defining characteristic occurs later than birth has members who have experienced risk of disease before they joined the cohort. Person time prior to becoming eligible for a study is an example of what is called *immortal person-time*. The term derives from the logical impossibility of death having occurred prior to the study for anybody included in the study. Immortal person-time should never be counted as part of the denominator of a rate calculation.

**Immortal person-time.** *The experience of study subjects that is event-free by definition is immortal person-time.*

When the Mt. Sinai researchers established a cohort of insulation workers who were union members on January 2, 1967 (Example 5.2), all prior experience of those men was immortal person-time, immortal because their presence in the cohort meant that they had not died earlier. Correctly, the researchers did not incorporate that past time into the person years recorded in Table 5.2.

Be aware that there is a distinction between the passage of time that must be accounted for in order to categorize an exposure correctly, and the passage of time that constitutes observed experience. The 15 years that had to elapse after first exposure to asbestos before a worker's person-time could appear in Table 4.2 were immortal person-time. Nonetheless, the time interval had to be accounted for in order to classify the observed person time. The first ten months of employment of the workers in Example 4.3 comprised immortal person-time.

When the observable person-time lies entirely outside the bounds of cohort membership, as in the insulation workers example, then it is easy to ignore the immortal person-time: it is inaccessible to direct observation. Similary, when accessible person-time has been excluded from an analysis, as were the very young and very old person-years of Table 4.3, the person time is effectively rendered immortal, but in an innocuous way. The threat posed by immortal person time arises only when it is included in the analysis.

Occasionally, a circumstance that defines exposure and cohort membership occurs in persons already under observation. For a study of the relation between replacement estrogen use and myocardial infarction in an HMO that had records of drug use and hospitalization, one might define a cohort of estrogen users who had not suffered a past MI. Women who were members of the HMO and who had not suffered an MI would enter the cohort at the time of first estrogen use, and their rate of occurrence of MI would be compared to a selected group of nonusers who had not suffered an MI at the beginning of the observation period. How should we allocate the person time at risk that the users accrued prior to their first pre-scription for replacement estrogens?

If the time were assigned to the "user" category, the effect would be to dilute the true person-time at risk among users with time during which no estrogens had been consumed. The result would evidently distort any apparent estrogen effect. Yet if the time were assigned to the nonuser category, there would also be a dilution: it is known a priori that no MI occurred during this time; women who had suffered an MI would never have entered the exposed cohort, and would not have come into our ken.

Segregate the time into a "pre-use" category and the correct analysis becomes obvious. The rate of MI prior to estrogen use in women chosen as being MI-free at the time of onset of estrogen use is necessarily zero. The time is immortal person-time and should be excluded from analysis.

A common feature of immortal person-time is that it occurs in study subjects prior to the events that designate them as being eligible for the study. Consider a variation on the example above. If the person time of all female members of the HMO who had not suffered an MI were being monitored and a woman who was a nonuser of replacement estrogens suffered an MI, and then subsequently used replacement estrogens, her person time prior to use (prior to the MI) would be legitimately counted in the category of "nonuser." The difference between this and the preceding example is that observation of the woman in this case is not contingent on her use of replacement estrogens. Note also that a nonfatal MI in this case marks the beginning of another sort of immortal person-time: we can never again observe a first time myocardial infarction.

# 5

# Cohort Studies

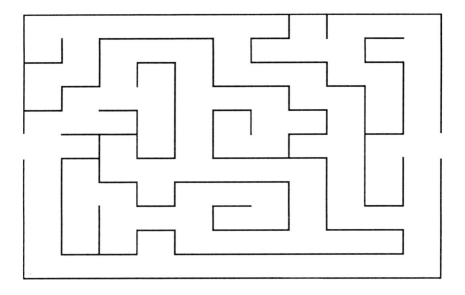

A population of known size, an elapse of time, the dates of onset: these are the necessary elements for quantifying the rate of occurrence of disease. In *closed cohort studies*, study subjects are observed continuously from the time of joining the study forward. "Exposure" is a state or characteristic present at the outset, and disease occurrences are accumulated to the end of follow-up. In *open cohort studies* there remains the key element of comparison of attained states (of exposure or of life style, for example), but the onset of the relevant state may lie outside the period of observation. *Case-control studies*, a special class of cohort studies in which the source population is studied on a sample basis, will be treated in the next chapter.

## Closed Cohort Studies

Consider an example from infectious disease epidemiology.

**Example 5.1.** *Foodborne streptococcal pharyngitis.*[45]

During June 21-24, 1979, 300 Greek-Americans held a convention in Palm Beach. There was an outbreak of pharyngitis during the convention. Fearing Legionnaire's Disease, local officials called on the United States Centers for Disease Control (CDC). Through interviews and mailed questionnaires, a CDC team attempted to identify the foods eaten and events attended by every conventioneer, and to define the time of onset of symptoms of pharyngitis. Cases of "convention-associated" pharyngitis were defined as any sore throat in a conventioneer that developed after arrival at the convention but before June 29. Because the study took place after the convention was over, it was possible to obtain throat cultures only from those conventioneers whose homes were near Palm Beach. Cultures were taken from both symptomatic and asymptomatic subjects, and cases in which there was a positive culture for Lancefield group G streptococci were classed as "culture-confirmed."

Populations at risk among the conventioneers were defined according to activities undertaken, and the risk of developing pharyngitis was calculated for each population defined by participation in a particular activity. After some preliminary review of the data, the investigators focused their attention on two events: a luncheon on June 22 and a dance held that same evening. It was possible to classify 226 people according to their attendance at the luncheon and the dance, and according to their later pharyngitis, as shown in Table 5.1.

Two of eight waiters and one of five cooks for the luncheon also developed pharyngitis. On the evening before the luncheon the cook who became ill had prepared a chicken salad consumed by essentially all those who partook of the meal. She later had a throat culture positive for group G streptococcus. Of 20 throat culture isolates of beta-hemolytic streptococci obtained by the CDC from symptomatic conventioneers, 17 were group G. The CDC investigators concluded that there had been an outbreak of foodborne group G streptococcal pharyngitis, probably with the

45. Stryker WS, Fraser CW, Facklam RR. Foodborne outbreak of group G streptococcal pharyngitis. Am J Epidemiol 1982;116:533-40

**Table 5.1** Cumulative incidence of pharyngitis in relation to attendance at the luncheon and the dance

| Luncheon | Dance | Number | Cases | Percent ill |
|----------|-------|--------|-------|-------------|
| No | No | 40 | 1 | 3 % |
| No | Yes | 77 | 11 | 14 % |
| Yes | No | 23 | 8 | 35 % |
| Yes | Yes | 86 | 47 | 55 % |

chicken salad as the common vehicle of exposure. They did not feel that they had a satisfactory explanation for the apparent association of disease with attendance at the dance.

This example differs little in form from problems that might be encountered in the study of cancer, AIDS, or myocardial infarction. Researchers who work with infectious diseases have access to prior bacteriologic knowledge that enables them to focus their inquiry, but the questions they encounter are very much like those that appear in cohort studies of all kinds.

*Definition of populations at risk.* The population targeted for investigation consisted of a fully enumerated group of individuals (persons who attended the convention), whose experience was under study for an explicit period of time (June 21 to 29, 1979). Subcohorts for comparison were defined by having achieved some state (the states of having attended the luncheon or the dance), and for those subcohorts the study began as of the time they achieved the states (after the dance on June 22). Note that the state defining the cohorts is not exposure to group G streptococcus, which is not known or even knowable for the entire population; the defining state is rather participation in an activity, such as attendance at the dance or luncheon; the activity is a correlate of the suspected source of disease.

The persons studied did not consist of all those who attended the convention, but rather those for whom it was possible to obtain data. (Table 5.1 accounts for only 75 percent of the conventioneers.) If a person's willingness to participate in this study were affected by whether or not he developed a sore throat, the apparent overall attack rates would be distorted. If willingness to participate depended on both sore throat and attendance at the dance or the luncheon (as might be the case if conventioneers had specific hypotheses about the origin of their illness), then the relations between events attended and disease could be distorted as well.

*Definition of disease outcomes.* "Convention-associated" pharyngitis was given an operational definition for the purposes of epidemiologic study; it was not the idealized (and observable) event causally linked to a particular bacterial exposure at the convention. A few cases actually due to the contamination of the chicken salad may not have been manifest by June 29; almost certainly, some of the cases that appeared after June 22 and before June 29 had no link with any of the events at the convention. In the absence of a way to distinguish those cases that were part of the epidemic from those that were coincidental, the CDC group invoked a temporal criterion whose purpose was to include as many of the truly epidemic cases and as few of the background cases as possible.

Time definitions of case eligibility and of cohort observation are logically interchangeable. If they are not identical, then there is a contradiction implicit in the study design. The specification of the population at risk immediately defines in part the eligible cases: they must have been members of the population when they became ill. In an analogous manner, disease definition carries an implicit definition of the population at risk. Thus the choice of June 29 as the last allowable day for the onset of a "convention-associated" pharyngitis delimited the effective period of observation of the cohorts.

In the same way that temporal definitions of disease status and cohort membership must be congruent, so must other aspects of case definition. The entity actually recorded in Table 5.1 is "sore throat"; attribution of the epidemic to group G streptococcal disease is the result of intensive study of a nonrandom subsample of the population. Had the CDC investigators insisted on culture-proven streptococcal infection as a defining characteristic of a case, they would have in effect reduced the cohorts under study to those in whom a throat culture was taken. Since persons not cultured could not possibly have been termed cases (no matter what their actual disease experience), then they would not have been members of the cohort under study.

Restriction of eligible cases to those with culture-proven disease would have led to a tractable problem of cohort definition in this example because there is little ambiguity as to who was given an opportunity for diagnosis. The situation may be less clear in investigations of chronic diseases that might be diagnosed only through procedures that are not in widespread use. For example, if one were to insist on a full autopsy for case definition in a study of cancer, then the population under investigation would really consist of all those persons in the cohort who would have had an autopsy, had they died with cancer. Ascertaining cohort membership on the basis of a condition that is not manifest is logically acceptable, but poses practical problems. In effect we are left to study not the occurrence of disease, but the occurrence of disease-plus-diagnosis. If exposure is a determinant of the performance of necessary diagnostic procedures, then exposure will be a determinant of diagnosed disease, even if it bears no causal relation to disease itself.

Correct diagnosis of disease is crucial to epidemiologic study, yet it appears that in some cases the determinants of diagnostic procedures may masquerade as determinants of disease. This happens when a "definitive" diagnostic maneuver is rarely performed. In such circumstances the epidemiologic definition of disease must be refocussed on ascertainable outcomes such as "sore throat," "sudden death," or "wasting and diarrhea." The relation between these observables and the diseases that they might be taken to represent, group G pharyngitis, ventricular fibrillation, or AIDS, respectively may need to be the object of a separate investigation if the connection is at all in doubt. When diagnostic opportunity is very widespread, the benefits conferred by the use of a rigorous case definition most often outweigh the distortion introduced by selective access.

**Open Cohort Studies**

In the preceding example, there were two elements of the study which were assumed to have a simple structure: a single disease risk was to be estimated for each exposure, and the populations under study were taken to be closed as to membership. Neither simplicity of the relation of risk to time, nor the integrity of populations under study carries over to studies of most chronic diseases, in which the pace of time is measured in years rather than days.

Because time affects risks and changes people, the unit of observation in studies of chronic disease shifts away from the individual and toward a quantum of experience that incorporates both individual identity and the passage of time. An individual's person time is measured by the length of time during which that individual resides in a (more or less) homogeneous state of risk, and is characterized according to categories derived from the subject's prior history. The typical unit of person time in cancer epidemiology is the "person year"; in the study of vaccine reactions it might be the "person day." The time units are interconvertible: one person year equals 365.25 person days. The usual convention for recording person time is to select the largest time unit over which changes in the risk under study are negligibly small.

*Collection and categorization of data in studies of person time.* For each homogeneous period of risk in a study subject's life, the researcher notes the duration and adds that amount of person time to a category based on the individual's past and current experience. Since an individual's past evolves with time, his life experience may contribute sequentially to many categories of person time. He ages, he suffers new exposures, he accumulates perhaps larger and larger amounts of past exposures. Each new category of experience is segregated and its duration added to the summed durations of experience of other people in similar circumstances.

The investigator accumulates a table of person years experienced by study subjects, cross-classified by the factors (such as age, sex, exposure, and calendar year) considered relevant to the occurrence of disease. At the same time, the investigator builds a parallel table of counts of events (disease onsets) under study; each event is assigned to a cell in the table of events that corresponds to the exact category of person time within which the event took place.

Ideally, the categories tabulated represent pools of human experience that are homogeneous insofar as the expected incidence rate of disease is concerned. Most incidence rates evolve continuously over time, however, and no system of cut-points to distinguish categories is entirely satisfactory. The conventions most often used represent a balance between conflicting demands of detail in the description of risk (which would require many narrowly defined categories) and precision in each of the category-specific estimates (which may require many person years of experience in each category and therefore lead to more encompassing boundaries). Typical cut-points in chronic disease studies are five-year groups of age, of duration of exposure, of time since exposure, or of calendar year of observation.  No "typical" convention should be adopted, however, unless the investigator is satisfied that the expectation of a nearly homogeneous incidence rate within each category is approximately correct.

The following example illustrates the construction of the data for a cohort study of cancer mortality.

**Example 5.2.**  *Lung cancer in asbestos workers.*[46]

For a study of the effects of asbestos exposure, some 17,800 members of the Union of Heat and Frost Insulation Workers were registered on January 2, 1967, with information obtained on their dates of birth and entry into the union.  This latter date was taken as the date of first exposure to large quantities of asbestos-containing products.  All deaths in union members (active or retired) were reported through the union to researchers, who sought both the death certificates and all available medical data on each of the decedents in order to characterize the cause of death.  The number of man years of observation in five-year categories of time since first exposure and of age were tabulated for the full membership, and each death was assigned to that category to which the union member was contributing person time of experience at the time of his death.

Table 5.2 presents an extract of the information acquired through this study in the course of the first ten years of data collection.  For each time interval listed in the first column, the second column shows the number of men who contributed some amount of person time to that category.  In the third column, the sums of the individual contributions to person time in each category are listed, and in the next column are the numbers of deaths from lung cancer observed in each category.  The last column gives the lung cancer mortality rate per 1000 person years, obtained by dividing the number of deaths from lung cancer in each category by the accumulated person years (measured in thousands) for the same category.

46. Selikoff IJ, Hammond EC, Seidman H.  Latency of asbestos disease among insulation workers in the United States and Canada. Cancer 1980;46:2736-40.

**Table 5.2**  Lung cancer mortality and time since onset of exposure to asbestos

| Time since first exposure (years) | Number of men who contributed experience | Person years of experience | Deaths from lung cancer | Deaths per 1000 person years |
|---|---|---|---|---|
| 15 - 19 | 9948 | 34,066 | 27 | 0.79 |
| 20 - 24 | 8887 | 31,268 | 57 | 1.82 |
| 25 - 29 | 6596 | 20,657 | 96 | 4.64 |
| 30 - 34 | 3547 | 11,598 | 103 | 8.88 |
| 35 - 39 | 2020 | 5,403 | 57 | 10.55 |
| 40 - 44 | 1108 | 3,160 | 31 | 9.81 |

Several features of Table 5.2 underscore the point that person time, not persons, is the object of classification and study. (1) The sum of the second column exceeds the total number of men observed in the study, because most men contributed to more than one category of time since first exposure. (2) Men who died of lung cancer contributed person time of experience both to the category that they were in when they died and to any previous category during which they had been observed. The person time at risk in a cohort study is contributed by those who later suffer an event as well as by those who never do. (3) Comparisons between any pair of mortality rates in Table 5.2 may involve the experience of some individuals who contribute to both exposure categories. By contrast, all comparisons in Table 5.1 necessarily involved separate individuals.

The mortality rates listed in the last column of Table 5.2 are examples of the fundamental epidemiologic measure offered by an open cohort study. From the pattern of mortality rates shown, it is evident that the lung cancer mortality rate rose dramatically with the passage of time from first exposure to asbestos, and that there was a plateau beginning after some 35 years. A deceleration in the rise of lung cancer rates after many years appears to be a nearly constant feature of cohorts of asbestos workers followed for the long term.[47] The relative mortality rates, as compared to the rates in the general population, actually tend to decline.

47. Walker AM. Declining relative risks for lung cancer after cessation of asbestos exposure. J Occup Med 1984;26:422-6

# 6

# Case-Control Studies

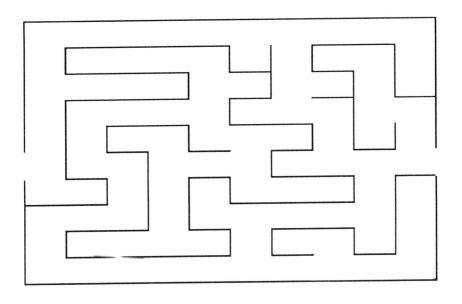

Case-control studies constitute the major advance in epidemiologic methods of our time. In itself the case-control study has greatly improved the efficiency of research into the etiology of rare conditions. Since the case-control study differs from the cohort study only in that knowledge about the source population is garnered through sampling, elucidation of the case-control study has also shed light on many subtleties of the parent design. I will develop the notation here for the case of sampling from open cohorts whose experience is measured in person time. There is a precisely analogous line of argument for case-control sampling from closed cohorts. Since everything that follows is predicated on the notion of sampling from an underlying cohort, essentially all the terminology, definitions, and caveats that apply to the conduct of research in cohorts will apply to case-control investigations as well.

## Case-Control Studies and the Cohorts that Underlie Them

Consider an open population with person time experience accumulating in two pools, which we will designate for convenience as "exposed" and "unexposed." Define the following quantities:

$P_1, P_0$    the accumulated person time in exposed and unexposed persons, respectively,

$x_1, x_0$    the corresponding observed numbers of cases,

$IR_1, IR_0$    the corresponding observed incidence rates of disease,

$RR$    the ratio of the observed incidence rate in exposed to that in unexposed persons.

The following relations exist among these various quantities:

$$IR_1 = \frac{x_1}{P_1}$$

$$IR_0 = \frac{x_0}{P_0}$$

$$RR = \frac{IR_1}{IR_0}$$

$$RR = \frac{x_1}{P_1} \Big/ \frac{x_0}{P_0}$$

$$RR = \frac{x_1}{x_0} \Big/ \frac{P_1}{P_0}$$

If the quantities $P_1$, $P_0$, $x_1$, and $x_0$ are all known for a given population, then there is no obstacle to calculating the incidence rates $IR_1$ and $IR_0$ and therefore the rate ratio $RR$. However, the cost of actually identifying the exposure status of a large and changing population may be high. If the exposure status of members of the population is changing even as the members remain under observation, the technical obstacles to maintaining current data may be insurmountable, no matter what resources are available.

A way around this barrier lies in the last formulation given above for the rate ratio. Even if the population distribution of exposure is unknown, it will generally be possible to ascertain the exposure status of the $x_1 + x_0$ individuals who develop disease. This might be accomplished by interview, for example, or by hand review of individual exposure records. Given $x_1$ and $x_0$, the remaining quantity to be identified in order to calculate the rate ratio is $P_1/P_0$. If it were possible to estimate the relative amounts of person time in the exposed and unexposed portions of the population, then estimation of the rate ratio could follow immediately, even in the absence of full exposure information on the underlying population.

If an estimate of $P_1/P_0$ were obtained by a sampling procedure, then the result would be subject to random error, but it would be valid in that the accuracy of the process producing it would be limited only by the number of individuals sampled. A study based on enumeration of the cases of disease and on random sampling of the person time giving rise to those cases provides a consistent[48] estimate of the rate ratio.

**Sampling the Source Population**

Consider mesothelioma, a rare malignancy for which all or nearly all cases in individuals under the age of 65 might be referred to a cancer center. Imagine that a study is being conducted in a region in which there is a single facility that will receive essentially all the cases from the area immediately surrounding it and a number of cases from more distant places as well. The population giving rise to cases of mesothelioma seen in the facility consists of all persons who would have been referred there, had they developed disease. While this is a logically valid definition, it is not one that leads immediately to any specific sampling policy. How can we know that a healthy person not from the immediately surrounding area would have been referred?

Instead of searching for ingenious methods of identifying the population at risk of referral from outside the immediate area, the investigator can simplify the task of sampling by incorporating a population specification into the case definition. If cases for the study are restricted to those who are treated at the facility and who are residents of districts surrounding the facility, for whom the probability of referral is nearly 100 percent, then the population at risk is immediately identified as the population resident in those districts during the period of case accrual.

---

48. Estimates which can be expected to come arbitrarily close to a value of interest as the sample size increases are said to be "consistent."

Sampling a geographically defined population in order to obtain a control series can be entirely straightforward. In many places, it is possible to obtain a complete list of residents. In this case the sampling procedure is as follows.

(1) Select a date at random from the case accrual period.

(2) Select a person at random from the population list.

(3) If the subject selected was actually resident within the predetermined area as of the random date chosen for that particular subject, then the subject is accepted as a control for the case-control study as of the randomly sampled day.

(4) Repeat the above three steps until the desired number of controls has been chosen.

(5) Any information collected from cases that invokes the date of onset of illness as a reference point (such as "A year prior to your diagnosis, did you ... ?") is collected from controls with reference to the random point in time that constituted part of the control definition.

Recall that $P_0$ and $P_1$ represent person time rather than persons, and that this distinction is necessary for calculation of incidence rates. The double control selection process (choosing a random time point from the case accrual period and a random subject from the population under study) samples person time rather than people. It can be shown that the probability of any given person day's becoming an index day in the control series is equal to that of any other person day experienced by the source population. By extension, the probability of any individual's being selected as a control can be demonstrated to be proportional to the duration of time that the individual spends in the source population at risk.

The investigator repeats the control selection procedure until he has obtained the desired number of controls. In so doing he establishes a probability for each person day at risk in the study person-time[49] that it will be chosen for the control series. If we represent this control selection probability as

$f$     the probability of selecting a given person day from the person time at risk,

---

49. c.f. Figure 3.6.

then we can represent the number of controls obtained in a case-control study as an expected function of exposure. Define the numbers of exposed and unexposed controls as

$y_1$    the number of selected controls who are exposed on their designated index day,

$y_0$    the number of selected controls who are not exposed as of their designated index day.

The operational definition of $f$ is

$$f = \frac{y_1 + y_0}{P_1 + P_0}$$

Since $f$ is defined without respect to exposure status, it follows that the expected values of $y_1$ and $y_0$ are

$$E(y_1) = f P_1$$
$$E(y_0) = f P_0$$

from which it is possible to obtain an expression for the rate ratio as a function of case and control counts:

$$RR = \frac{x_1}{x_0} / \frac{P_1}{P_0}$$

$$= \frac{x_1}{x_0} / \frac{f P_1}{f P_0}$$

$$= \frac{x_1}{x_0} / \frac{E(y_1)}{E(y_0)}$$

Substitution of the observed for the expected counts yields the *odds ratio* of the table, which is an estimate of the incidence rate ratio

$$RR \doteq \frac{x_1 y_0}{y_1 x_0} = OR$$

The value $x_1/x_0$ is called the "exposure odds" for cases; $y_1/y_0$ is the exposure odds for controls. The term (like many concepts in statistics) is derived from gambling: the odds that a given case will be exposed are "$x_1$ to $x_0$". The rate ratio estimate in a case-control study is the ratio of the exposure odds in cases to the exposure odds in controls, and is therefore often called the "odds ratio."

**Example 6.1.** *Cryptorchidism and testicular cancer.*[50]

Morrison conducted a study of testicular cancer, using medical records kept by the United States Army. From a pathology index, he identified 596 cases of testicular cancer among soldiers, and he noted the date of diagnosis of each. He then established a scheme for locating comparison records at random: for research purposes there had already been developed a list consisting of one tenth of one percent of military personnel who were active during the time of the study. Using the last digits of the soldiers' military identification numbers, Morrison obtained a subsample of this research list to serve as comparison subjects (controls). He reviewed the physical examinations carried out at the time of induction into the army of the testicular cancer patients (the cases) and 602 controls in order to establish the prevalence of treated or untreated undescended testis in each group. Since the exposure under study did not vary with time (and presumably did not affect duration of service in the army), Morrison did not need to make provision for a single date as of which to define the exposure status of controls. He obtained the data of Table 6.1.

**Table 6.1** Cryptorchidism and testicular cancer in the U.S. Army

|                  | Cryptorchid | Not cryptorchid |
|------------------|:-----------:|:---------------:|
| Testicular cancer |     17      |       579       |
| Controls          |      2      |       600       |

$$RR = \frac{(17)(600)}{(2)(579)} = 8.8$$

50. Morrison AS. Cryptorchidism, hernia, and cancer of the testis. J Natl Cancer Inst 1976;56:731-3

## Pseudo-Sampling When the Source Population is not Identified

It may happen that there is no ready list of persons in the source population, nor even a list of some larger population from which the desired population members might be culled. In the preceding example, if there were two oncology centers serving the same region, then the referral of patients to one or the other center might be the result of a series of seemingly haphazard events related to the choice of physician, the presence of relatives near one center, and so forth. We cannot know exactly who those persons are who would have been referred, much less sample them. One frequently chosen solution is to select controls from those persons who were in fact referred to the oncology center that provides our cases. The date of disease that defines controls is taken as each control's index date. Controls so chosen must have diseases unrelated to the exposures under study.

Denote the incidence rate of a comparison disease by $Q$. Suppose that, within categories of all the ascertained characteristics of study subjects other than exposure, the comparison disease incidence rate is identical in persons with and without the exposures under study. Imagine furthermore that the referral patterns for the comparison disease and for the primary disease under study are identical. If the persons with the comparison disease are taken as controls, then the expected number of exposed and unexposed controls taken together is

$$E(y_1 + y_0) = Q(P_1 + P_0)$$

and since incidence is unrelated to exposure status,

$$E(y_1) = QP_1$$
$$E(y_0) = QP_0$$

From here the argument leading to the odds ratio as an estimate of the rate ratio proceeds exactly as before, except that $Q$, the incidence rate of the comparison disease, takes the place of $f$, the probability of selecting a given control day out of the person time at risk. Although there is no theoretical difficulty in utilizing diseased controls, there are practical problems in assuring the validity of the assumptions that underlie the practice. Is $Q$, the incidence rate of the comparison disease, unrelated to the exposures under study in the source population? A valid case-control analysis assumes not that there is no causal association between exposure and the comparison disease, but that there is no variation *for any reason* in the comparison disease incidence rate across categories of exposure.

To some extent, the validity of the comparison series may be examined by choosing a number of disease entities for inclusion. If each truly portrays exposure in the source population, then each of the comparison entities ought to provide similar estimates of exposure prevalence, up to whatever level of accuracy is imposed by chance variation. Thus the various control diseases can be compared in terms of their exposure prevalence. If there are any outliers, these groups are removed on the presumption that they are biased with respect to exposure for some previously unsuspected reason. If no group's exposure experience is dissimilar to that of the others, then the hypothesis that each is a valid representation of exposure patterns in the base population is strengthened. All of the control groups are then collapsed together for the purposes of analysis.

The use of diseased controls brings up considerations peculiar to the medical facilities in which the cases and controls are ascertained. Are the probabilities of diagnosis and referral to the facility generating the cases identical for the comparison disease and the disease under study? If not, then the source population for controls differs from that for cases; the validity of the control series depends on a further assumption of homology between the source population for cases and that for controls. If the prevalence of exposure in the control source population is identical to that in the case source population, and if $Q$, the incidence of the control disease, is unrelated to exposure in the source population for controls, then the control series provides an unbiased estimate of exposure prevalence in the source population for cases, and the odds ratio estimate of the rate ratio is valid. The practice of comparing exposure prevalence in different control groups, noted above, does not provide strong evidence of the suitability of controls whose source population differs from that of the cases.

**Clinical Aspects of Case Definition**

As in cohort studies, the criteria for case definition in a case-control study depend on the amount of information routinely available on potential cases within the source population. While investigators may sometimes establish a dedicated surveillance network to detect all potential cases, it is much more common for epidemiologic research to depend on routinely collected data. In this latter circumstance, the investigator balances a desire for accuracy in case designation against the danger of obtaining a case series in which principal determinants of case status are the social or demographic determinants of diagnosis. An optimal case definition depends on criteria that can be applied to any potential case in the source population.

An epidemiologic study is at high risk of detecting spurious associations whenever case definition depends on a diagnostic procedure that is rarely performed, such as autopsy, or on the judgment of specialists. Most psychiatric disorders fall into the latter category, and Alzheimer's Disease would be an example of the former. By the same token, studies of generally benign conditions run a high risk of mistaking correlates of easy access to medical care for etiologic factors. Functional ovarian cysts and gallstones would be two examples: in each case there is a high prevalence of a mildly symptomatic disease whose diagnosis *may* occur in persons who consult physicians often for other reasons, but will not occur otherwise.

Note how very different are the roles of case ascertainment in an epidemiologic study and in a clinical therapeutic trial. In the clinical trial, where the goal is to evaluate the efficacy of therapy, the overriding concern is that subjects entered into the trial actually have the disease in question. Those excluded from the trial are of no interest. In an epidemiologic study the focus is on the relative frequency with which persons with different exposure statuses develop disease. Factors that lead to the exclusion of true cases are of concern, particularly if correlated with exposure. If case definition requires the use of diagnostic procedures that cannot be made uniformly available, then it may be that the population in question is not a suitable starting point for the conduct of a case-control study.

Almost as important as identifying cases correctly is the specification of a time at which the individuals in question undergo the transition from "healthy" to "ill." This is the case for two reasons. First, any comprehensible discussion of exposures that change with time or of exposure effects that change with time requires unambiguous definitions of those times at which the exposures (or their residua) are considered to be acting. Second, exposures measured after the onset of illness may provide a poor stand-in for earlier exposures, particularly when disease affects lifestyle or work patterns.

Seldom is it possible to identify the onset of a chronic disease, and the solutions that have been applied to the problem have a disconcerting, *ad hoc* quality. Occasionally researchers estimate presumed times of onset on the basis of (untestable) assumptions about the rate of progression from incipient to clinical stages of illness. For diseases that generally lead to a hospitalization, it is common simply to establish the date of first diagnosis or the date of first hospitalization leading to a diagnosis as an index date. Questions about exposures that might be affected by disease are backdated to an index date that precedes most durations of symptoms prior to onset, as determined clinically.

Vigorous pursuit of efforts at backdating disease onset frequently raises more problems than are resolved. An estimated date of onset far into the past may locate the disease event in a source population that cannot be properly sampled. An unobserved date of presumed onset that precedes case identification may raise the possibility of cases to be identified in the future that will be ascribed to the current study time: factors that lead to early detection can then masquerade as predictors of the disease. The best solution is to identify incidence-dates that are closely tied to events observable in all members of the source population. Then be clear that you are studying what has been defined, and separately speculate on or investigate the relation between the operational criterion and the imagined true event.

### Alternatives to Simple Causal Interpretation

It often happens that there is some extra characteristic of individuals in the study population (beyond exposure and disease) that threatens to distort the apparent exposure-disease relation. This situation occurs when the extra factor is itself a predictor of disease risk and is not evenly distributed between the exposed and unexposed sectors of the population. An evaluation of the occurrence of disease according to exposure is then contaminated by the different expectations of disease occurrence in the exposed and unexposed groups, even in the absence of an effect of exposure itself. As in the analysis of cohort data, the admixture of an extraneous effect in the comparison of two exposure groups in a case-control study is called *confounding*. The presence of confounding is a characteristic of the population and disease under study, and it poses the same threat to validity in case-control studies that it does in cohort studies.

Just as in the analysis of cohort studies, the most common solution to the problem of confounding is to segregate study subjects into subgroups, or strata, within which there is little or no variation in the extent of the extra factor, the predictor of disease that threatens to confound the unstratified ("crude") analysis. After stratification, there is little or no residual potential for confounding within each stratum. By definition, the third factor is identical in exposed and unexposed persons within each stratum.

For any observational study, the search for confounding factors amounts to a search for alternative causal explanations for an observed exposure-disease relation. In those case-control studies in which it has been impossible to obtain for the control series a simple random sample of the population giving rise to the cases, it is imperative to ask whether or not the factors determining control selection are likely to have yielded a comparison group whose relevant exposure characteristics accurately reflect those of the source population for cases.

**Example 6.2.** *Ferruginous bodies and lung cancer.*[51]

Warnock and Churg sought to evaluate the effects of low level asbestos exposure in the production of bronchogenic carcinoma of the lung through a case-control study. Their measure of low level exposure was based on an analysis of the concentration of a marker of cumulative asbestos exposure, ferruginous bodies (also called "asbestos bodies"), in lung tissue. The cases were 30 persons who had died with lung cancer; ferruginous body counts were carried out *post mortem*. Since Warnock and Churg could not directly measure ferruginous bodies in the lungs of persons in the population giving rise to the lung cancer cases, they performed similar measurements on 100 consecutive autopsies of persons over the age of 20 during a period that encompassed the accrual of lung cancer cases. The results of the analysis, shown in Table 6.2, indicate nearly a seven fold elevation of lung cancer mortality in persons with low-level exposure.

For the relation between ferruginous bodies and lung cancer, the strength of the association noted above would raise a warning signal to anyone familiar with the subsequent literature on the relation between asbestos and pulmonary disease. A relative mortality on the

---

51. Warnock ML, Churg AM. Association of asbestos and bronchogenic carcinoma in a population with low asbestos exposure. Cancer 1975;35:1236-42

**Table 6.2** Lung cancer and ferruginous bodies in lung tissue

|                | Bodies per gram of wet tissue | |
|----------------|:---------:|:---------:|
|                | $\geq 50$ | $< 50$ |
| Lung cancer    | 8         | 22        |
| Other          | 5         | 95        |

$$RR = \frac{(8)(95)}{(22)(5)} = 6.9$$

order of five has been observed for lung cancer in some (but by no means all) cohorts of workers heavily exposed to asbestos throughout their lifetimes. That a similar risk should obtain for the subset of the general population with low-to-moderate asbestos exposure seems improbable.

Several distortions are evident. The first is related to cigarette smoking. Tobacco is a potent inducer of bronchogenic carcinoma. Cigarette smoking in the United States during the period of study was related to social class, with laborers smoking more than white collar workers. As a result there existed an association between on-the-job asbestos exposure and smoking whose basis was entirely sociological. Connected to both exposure and risk of disease, tobacco use might then be expected to confound the apparent relation between the two. There may also be a selective distortion of the data (sometimes called "information bias"). Smokers suffer paralysis of the bronchial cilia responsible for clearing mucus, and are thus likely to retain for a longer time inhaled particulates, including asbestos fibers, which can give rise to ferruginous bodies. The measure of asbestos exposure itself, the concentration of ferruginous bodies in lung tissue, may therefore have been exaggerated by concomitant use of cigarettes. Whether exaggeration of the measure (ferruginous bodies) reflects an increase in the relevant carcinogenic exposure is a matter of speculation: the properties of asbestos that result in carcinogenicity are not well understood.

Age in this example carries a clear potential for confounding, in that it is related to both mortality from lung cancer (which rises as the fourth or fifth power of age) and to the accumulation of ferruginous bodies in lung tissue (as a more or less linear function of age for environmental asbestos pollution). A comparison of lung cancer cases with a true random sample from the general population would yield a very strong association between ferruginous body levels and disease, on the basis of age confounding alone. To an unknown extent this distortion has been reduced by the use of dead controls, who are more likely to have had the age distribution of lung cancer cases than did the population at large.

A comparison of lung cancer victims with other decedents depends on the assumption that exposure to low levels of asbestos does not appreciably affect mortality from causes other than lung cancer. On the basis of other studies, this seems to be a reasonable hypothesis. Warnock and Churg also presumed that differences in the source populations for cases and controls as well as the determinants of autopsy were unrelated to pulmonary ferruginous body concentrations. Since the exposure measurement was available only after autopsy, the decision to carry out the autopsy was almost certain not to have been related to the measure itself. However, there is a strong possibility that cases of different complexity (and therefore different likelihood of undergoing autopsy) derive from referral areas that are not coextensive. As ambient asbestos levels vary with locale, it is not at all obvious that the controls provide information on the precise population from which the cases were drawn. Since this latter source population has remained unspecified in the study design, there is no opportunity for further evaluation of the bias.

# 7

# Generalization

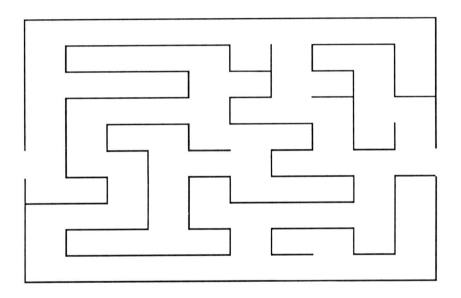

The purpose of this chapter is to introduce the vocabulary used to link theory and observations. Parameters are theoretical values; they determine the shape and location of the long-range frequency distributions for observed data. Two parameters will be discussed: probability, which characterizes both prevalences and cumulative incidences, and hazard, which characterizes incidence rates. Both statistical and systematic errors in parameter estimates will be addressed. Confounding is an example of systematic error that arises when a planned comparison juxtaposes noncomparable groups. There is also the uncomfortable, empirical fact that epidemiologic observations are less fully replicable than statistical models suggest they ought to be.

## Parameters

While rare exposures, such as standing at ground zero of a hydrogen blast, may absolutely determine vital status, most determinants of health are accompanied by an element of uncertainty. Even very similar individuals (identical twins, for example), do not have precisely the same health status throughout their lives.

A deterministic view of disease causation can account for uncertainty about the cumulative incidence for any particular group by holding that study groups are the imperfect reflection of an underlying reality. The "reality" is envisioned as the class of all possible subjects meeting study criteria, and the studied property of that infinite class is the proportion destined, for example, to have a heart attack within a year. If the presence of that characteristic is unknown on an individual level, then the proportion that characterizes the class can differ from the observed cumulative incidence because of vagaries in the selection of the study population. The class feature that the observed data approximate, the overall proportion in the imagined class of similar individuals, is referred to as the *probability* of disease.

A probabilistic view of disease causation postulates an unknown mechanism operating within individuals, a black box, that behaves as if governed by a random process with stable long-term characteristics. The long-term fraction of persons who manifest disease is the probability that characterizes the process. Chance here is only a metaphor for the true mechanism of disease production, just as it is only a metaphor for the process of subject selection from an imaginary universe of all possible subjects in the preceding view.

For the purposes of inference from observation to the underlying reality, the arguments presented later will assume that there is a general characteristic of the process giving rise to disease in a particular study group that can be meaningfully summarized as a single number between zero and one, inclusive.

**Probability** *is a characteristic of the physical processes that give rise to observable events, and represents the limiting value that would be observed for a cumulative incidence or a prevalence as larger and larger numbers of individuals came under scrutiny.*[52]

---

52. "Risk" is a synonym for probability.

The true probability of an event in an individual is either one or zero for a determinist, and the 20 percent that might be estimated from group data is a measure of the determinist's degree of belief that any one of the individuals who comprise the group actually possesses sufficient elements for the manifestation of disease. For a probabilist, who accepts the black box, the probability of disease in an individual is the expected value of the cumulative incidence in essentially similar persons.

The probability of an event is a *parameter*, the procedure for obtaining a cumulative incidence is an *estimator*, and the cumulative incidence calculated from a particular set of data is an *estimate* of the probability.

**Parameter.** *The terms other than those describing the circumstances of observation and the outcome in the formulaic presentation of a probability distribution are parameters. Parameters are not observable, but may be estimated from observations.*

**Estimator.** *An estimator is a procedure for obtaining estimates. It is, equivalently, a random variable whose realization, the "estimate," will be taken as a measure of a parameter. The estimator is a function of random variables whose realizations are the data points being observed.*

**Estimate.** *An estimate is a realization of the estimator. The estimate is a function of the observed data.*

The following section will address the ways in which estimates provide information about parameters.

Probability serves the epidemiologist as the parameter corresponding to the prevalence of a characteristic or the cumulative incidence of disease; for the statistician, probability plays another role. In a hypothetical population of repeated identical studies, probability also describes the proportion of studies expected to have a particular outcome. "Statistical Uncertainty" (below) will speak to this aspect of probability.

In order to make the transition from the probability parameter to a parameter that corresponds to the incidence rate, we need to adopt some formalisms for the description of time and temporal relations. A bracket, "[" or "]", next to a time designation means that a starting or stopping time is included in the interval that it bounds. An ordinary parenthesis, "(" or ")", means that the time point is not included in the interval in question. Written symbolically, the interval that begins just after $t_1$ and continues through time $t_2$ is $(t_1,t_2]$, and the cumulative incidence, $CI$, over that interval is $CI(t_1,t_2]$. In the absence of loss to follow-up during $(t_1,t_2]$, the defining equation for the cumulative incidence is

$$CI(t_1,t_2] = \frac{\text{Cases}(t_1,t_2]}{N(t_1)}$$

$N(t_1)$ is the size of the population that is at risk to become an incident case at time $t_1$. Denote the probability of acquiring disease during the interval $(t_1,t_2]$ by $R(t_1,t_2]$. $CI$ is an estimate of $R$. Clearly, as $t_2$ gets closer to $t_1$, $R(t_1,t_2]$ approaches zero. However, by dividing $R(t_1,t_2]$ by the length of the time interval over which the cumulative incidence is calculated (obtained by subtracting $t_1$ from $t_2$), it is possible to obtain a stable, limiting value, characteristic of $t_1$, called the *hazard*, and denoted symbolically by $h$.

$$h(t_1) = \lim_{t_2 \to t_1} \frac{R(t_1,t_2]}{t_2 - t_1}$$

$$= \frac{dR(t_1,t_2]}{dt_2}\bigg|_{t_2 = t_1}$$

The symbol "$\lim_{t_2 \to t_1}$" means "the value approached as $t_2$ comes closer to $t_1$." The convention in the second line of the above equation describes incremental changes; "$dx/dy$" means "the incremental change in $x$ associated with each change in $y$." The vertical bar with the subscript "$t_2=t_1$" at the end of the expression means "evaluated when $t_2$ equals $t_1$," that is right at the beginning of follow-up. The second line thus refers to the incremental change in the probability of survival immediately following $t_1$. The incremental changes could be read as the slope at $t_2=t_1$ of a graph of $R(t_1,t_2]$ versus $t_2$.[53]

**Hazard.** *The hazard is the limiting value of the probability of becoming an incident case per unit time among those at risk for becoming a case.*

---

53. Look again at the daily incidence curve of Figure 1.3.

The hazard function has the units "change in the number of cases per population size ($N$) per unit time," so that the unit of measurement, or *dimension*, of a hazard is "cases per *person time*." The units of the daily incidence of bleeding shown in Figure 1.3 would be cases per person day.

The dimension of hazard as it appears in the literature of survival theory, and in some epidemiologic texts, is the reciprocal of time. The transition from "cases per person time" to "per time" is achieved by observing that "cases" are simply a count and therefore dimensionless, and that "person time" is a cumulation over persons of times observed in those persons, and therefore has the dimension of "time."

Defined as they have been above, hazards characterize instants. During short intervals, an insufficient number of events occurs to provide a useful estimate of hazard. Therefore, observations designed to permit an estimate of the hazard invoke the assumption that there are periods of time and population definitions that together can specify some finite quantity of person time during which, to a reasonable approximation, the hazard can be taken to be constant. Within such blocks of person time, an estimate of the hazard is provided by the incidence rate.

The relation between incidence rate and hazard is analogous to that between cumulative incidence and probability. The incidence rate is the observable counterpart of hazard. The hazard is the parameter of which the incidence rate is an estimator. The hazard is the value to which the incidence rate would tend as the amount of person time under observation became larger and larger. Refer again to Table 1.2.

### Statistical Uncertainty

When the observed data are precisely those that would be expected under a hypothesis that some particular parameter value is true, then we take that hypothesis as an estimate of the parameter. The concept of statistical uncertainty permits an extension of this procedure to statements about the consistency of data with parameters that predict something else, and even to situations in which the data observed would not have been expected under any single parameter. (This arises when different estimates of a single quantity disagree.) A good estimate will be a value that, if it were the parameter, would place the observed data in a position of highest possible probability. There is, however, no guarantee that such an estimate actually equals the estimated parameter.

The unknown distance that separates an estimate from its corresponding parameter raises the problem of statistical inference. Uncertain observations are compatible with an infinite number of parametric "truths," and one job of the statistician is to lay down limits on the kinds of realities that might have given rise to a set of data.

Figure 7.1 presents an idealized picture of the relative frequency of different estimates of a parameter whose true value has been taken for the purposes of illustration as 5. The curve is an example of a *probability density function*, and has a highly characteristic shape. The area under the curve is precisely one unit, and the probability that any particular estimate will fall between two values is equal to the area under the portion of the curve bounded by those values.

From inspection of Figure 7.1, it is evident that the greatest probabilities are associated with estimates near the true parameter value, and that the probability of estimates in an interval of any particular size falls off rapidly as the interval becomes removed from the true parameter value. The whole open-ended interval that begins 1.96 units above the parameter has an area of 0.025, indicating that such extreme values occur in about 2.5 percent of estimates. The curve is symmetrical, and the sum of the two tail areas that are bounded by 1.96 units above and below is five percent.

The units of the horizontal axis of Figure 7.1 are *standard errors*, and the shape of the curve is given by the so called *Normal* or *Gaussian* probability distribution. The curve, first described by Carl Friedrich Gauss to account for errors of measurement in astronomy, is the limiting form of the error distribution of all epidemiologic measures.

**Normal distribution**, *also called the Gaussian distribution, is the probability density function that describes the distribution of realizations x of a continuous random variable X when the value x is the sum of a very large number of random variables whose probability distribution is arbitrary, but whose variances (see below) are of similar magnitude.*

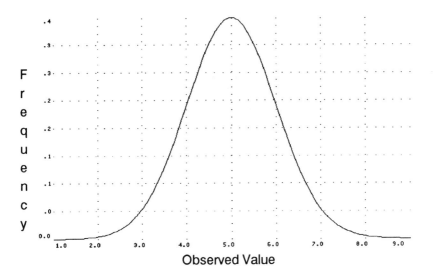

**Figure 7.1** Distribution of estimates of a hypothetical parameter

The standard error is the square root of the *variance*, a measure of the dispersion of a probability distribution. In order to assess the large sample properties of any estimator of a parameter, the analyst needs only the parameter value and the standard error of the estimator.

**Standard error.** *The standard error of an estimate is the square root of the variance of the estimator.*

**Variance.** *The variance of a random variable is the expected value of the square of the deviation of x from the expected value of X.*[54]

By one convention, estimates that fall more than 1.96 standard errors away from the parameter value are considered improbable (though they do occur five percent of the time). The importance of the convention is that it opens a path for inductive reasoning: begin with the observations and proceed to a statement about an unknown parameter. The trick is to hypothesize a parameter value, calculate the probability distribution of estimates under the hypothesis, and

---

54. See below and Chapter 13 for formal definitions of "expected value."

then to locate the known estimate on that distribution. If the estimate, which is known, would be improbable under the hypothesis represented by a particular parameter value, then the parameter value is *rejected* as a candidate explanation for the data.

Two widely used applications of this reasoning process are the *p value* and the *confidence interval*. The p (for probability) value is the tail area beyond the given estimate, assuming a particular parameter. The parameter assumed is most commonly one that represents a nil effect, and the p value is the probability of getting either the estimate actually obtained or an estimate further from the nil value. If this tail probability is low, and the hypothesis of a nil effect is rejected, then it follows that the effect must be non-nil. When the p value is less than some prespecified cutoff, such as five percent or one percent, then the estimate differs from the nil effect level by a *statistically significant* amount.

**p value.** *The p value is the probability of occurrence of estimates that are as or more deviant from posited parameter values than the estimates actually obtained from a body of data. The p value is a function of observed data. It is the realization of a random variable whose distribution is uniform in the range [0, 1] under posited parameter values, and whose distribution becomes non-uniform, with an increased density near zero, under specified kinds of deviation from the posited values.*

Confidence intervals provide a more exhaustive application of statistical inference. A range of acceptable parameter estimates can be derived as those for which the observed data would not be too improbable. For any estimate, two hypothetical parameter values, one below the estimate and the other above, are identified to meet the following criterion: the size of the tail area that the estimate cuts off from the probability distributions implied by each of the two hypothetical parameter values is some prespecified amount. The sum of the two tail areas conventionally is either five or ten percent. If the tail areas sum to five percent, then the interval between the hypothetical parameters is a *95 percent confidence interval*; if the tail areas sum to ten percent, then the interval is a 90 percent confidence interval.

**Confidence interval.** *A confidence interval is a set of possible parameter values that are consistent with a body of observations in the sense that the p values for the data given any of the parameter values in the interval are greater than a specified amount, usually* *designated by* α. *The salient operational feature of a confidence interval is that it is calculated by a mechanism that has a priori a* 1-α *probability of including the true parameter value.*

For the measures considered in this text, a large-sample 95 percent confidence interval can always be constructed as follows.

(1) Identify the standard error associated with a particular measure. This value is the square root of the variance of the measure, and is a function of the parameter being estimated and of the number and the characteristics of subjects studied.

(2) Calculate the distance separating a parameter from an estimate that corresponds to a tail area of 2.5 percent. The distance is 1.96 times the standard error.

(3) Add the calculated distance to the estimate to obtain the upper 95 percent confidence bound.

(4) Subtract the calculated distance from the estimate to obtain the lower 95 percent confidence bound.

The parameter values that lie within the 95 percent confidence interval constitute a set of possible realities that are consistent with the observed data.

The arbitrariness of a choice of 90 or 95 percent confidence should be evident. The utility of the interval is not explicitly to include or exclude parameter values of interest, but rather to provide an indication of the range of true values that may have given rise to a given set of study results. A number of examples of confidence interval calculations are given in Chapter 8.

**Confounding**

The analysis of random error presupposes that there is no difference between comparison groups such as might give rise to different disease frequencies, other than the factor that is used to define the groups. Even in a carefully designed study, there is no guarantee of this kind of comparability. The distortion of analytic results that can arise from dissimilar comparison groups is called *confounding.* Confounding produces an *expected value* of the estimate that is different from the value of the parameter being estimates. Confounding is a form of *bias.*

**Expected value.** *The expected value of a random variable X is the average value that is observed in many repeated realizations of X.*

**Confounding.** *When imbalances in the composition of compared groups give rise to an expected value of a comparative measure that differs from the effect of the factor that defines the groups, the estimate of the effect of that factor is said to be confounded.*

**Bias.** *The difference between the expected value of an estimator and the parameter whose value is being estimated is the bias of the estimator.*

The relation of confounding to the characteristics of the study population will be explored in a separate chapter. One proper way to deal with confounding by factors that can be measured is to separate the study groups according to levels of the confounding factor. This is the core of stratified analyses, which will be dealt with in Chapter 8. The anticipated magnitude of confounding in an analysis that ignores the confounding factor is the subject of Chapter 9.

The inclusion of the term "expected value" in the definition of confounding implies the existence of chance mechanisms that could lead to estimates not equal to the parameter value even in the absence of confounding. In a fully deterministic view of disease causation, the "chance" processes are unmeasured determinants of disease, and any net contribution of those factors to disease is a form of confounding.

### Uncertainty Missed by Statistical Models

In small studies, the estimated effects of chance may overwhelm errors arising from other sources, and the p values and confidence intervals calculated in standard ways may provide useful guides to the imprecision of estimates. This utility does not extend to large studies. Chance, with its estimable errors, is sadly not the principal source of invalidity in most observational research.

Compilations of estimates from multiple studies are undertaken with increasing frequency, and statistical uncertainty has been found regularly to understate interstudy variability, particularly when the numbers of observations have been sufficiently large as to reduce the statistical uncertainty to modest proportions. For this reason, inference based on statistical considerations alone gives a more optimistic picture of the precision of knowledge than the data really justify. The chief role for the confidence interval estimates found in Chapter 8 is to set an upper bound to the analyst's certainty about the meaning of the results in hand.

Strict determinism and probabilistic views of disease causation differ strikingly in the directions in which they look to resolve questions of residual uncertainty. The determinist, driven by the idea that the origins of every instance of illness are knowable, will pursue details of exposure and host characteristics that are so individual as to reduce epidemiology to case reports. By contrast, the probabilist's black box can be enlarged to any dimension, and he is disinclined to pursue population differences that he ascribes to chance. Although the latter view empirically seems associated with less time wasted in the pursuit of the unknowable, the former leads to most new understanding of causal relations: the specific well-documented instance becomes the paradigm for a previously unimagined class. In the area of medical statistics, the role of the determinist is most often adopted by the investigating clinician, that of the probabilist by the statistician. Epidemiologists, who may come out of either tradition, do best when they keep a foot in either camp.

# 8

# Estimation

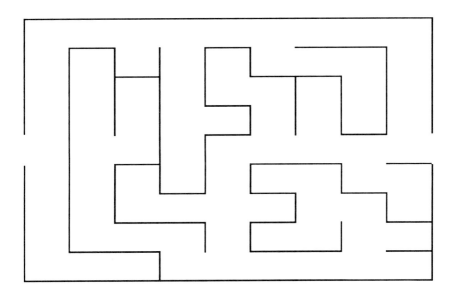

On the basis of data, we make estimates. The estimates are constructed in such a way that they bear a known relation to the parameters of processes that gave rise to the data. This chapter describes the mechanics of obtaining estimates and of judging the relation between estimate and parameter for closed and open cohort studies, and for case-control studies. All the statistical terms used here are defined in Chapter 13.

## Analysis of Closed Cohort Studies

The methods presented here will be illustrated using the data of Example 5.1, which you should review before continuing.

*Calculation of attack rates and cumulative incidence differences.* Since pharyngitis could only occur once during the period of observation, the designation of each of the cohort members as a case or non-case was unambiguous, and it was reasonable to calculate the fraction of persons in each cohort who became ill. This is the cumulative incidence, as defined in Chapter 1. Infectious disease epidemiology has its own term for the cumulative incidence: *attack rate (AR)*.[55]

**Attack rate.** *The attack rate is the cumulative incidence of disease in persons who are exposed to an agent whose effect is shorter than the time of potential follow-up. The period of follow-up begins at the time of exposure and continues over a closed interval that allows the expression of all possible new cases attributable to the exposure.*

The attack rate provides an estimate of the probability of infection that each of the cohort members faced at the beginning of the convention. Since the attack rate and the cumulative incidence are identical quantities, the latter term will be used in the remainder of this section for consistency. Readers should bear in mind that the infectious disease literature uses the former term. The cumulative incidence difference is obtained by subtracting the cumulative incidence in an unexposed group from that in an exposed group. Thus, in Table 5.1, the cumulative incidence difference associated with luncheon attendance is (47/86)-(11/77) or 40.4 percent in those who attended the dance and (8/23)-(1/40) or 32.3 percent in those who did not attend the dance.

Cumulative incidences and cumulative incidence differences observed in particular studies are estimates. Approximate confidence intervals for each of the corresponding probabilities and for their differences can be derived by assuming that the number of cases is distributed as a binomial variable.

---

55. The word "rate" in this term is a misnomer in the system of nomenclature presented here, since the attack rate is not a rate but a proportion.

**Binomial distribution** *is the probability distribution that describes the number of events observed in N opportunities to observe an event, when the probability of observing a single event at any opportunity is π, and is unaffected by the observation of an event at any other opportunity.*

$$\Pr(x \mid N) = \frac{N!}{x!(N-x)!} \pi^x (1-\pi)^{N-x}$$

$$E(X) = \pi N$$

$$\mathrm{Var}(X) = N\pi(1-\pi)$$

*The range of possible values for x is [0,N]. π is the binomial parameter.*

In this definition, as elsewhere, "Pr($x|N$)" means "the probability of observing $x$ cases among $N$ observed persons"; "E($X$)" means "the expected value of the random variable $X$"; and "Var($X$)" means "the variance of the random variable $X$."

In the calculation of a cumulative incidence, $x$ is the number of cases and $N$ is the number of individuals in the population at risk; the cumulative incidence is given by $x/N$. The variance of $x/N$ is $x(N-x)/N^3$.[56] The bounds of an approximate 95 percent confidence interval for the probability of pharyngitis, of which $x/N$ is an estimate, are obtained by adding and subtracting 1.96 times the standard error (the square root of the variance) to and from $x/N$. For those who attended the luncheon and the dance, $x$ is 47 and $N$ is 86, so that

$$CI = AR = x/N = 47/86 = 0.547$$

The 95 percent confidence bounds for the probability of pharyngitis are

---

56. c.f. Table 1.2 and Chapter 13. Note that

$$CI = \frac{x}{N}$$

$$\frac{CI(1-CI)}{N} = \frac{x(N-x)}{N^3}$$

$$\text{lower} = \frac{x}{N} - 1.96 \sqrt{\frac{x(N-x)}{N^3}}$$

$$= \frac{47}{86} - 1.96 \sqrt{\frac{47(86-47)}{86^3}}$$

$$= 0.441$$

$$\text{upper} = \frac{x}{N} + 1.96 \sqrt{\frac{x(N-x)}{N^3}}$$

$$= \frac{47}{86} + 1.96 \sqrt{\frac{47(86-47)}{86^3}}$$

$$= 0.652$$

The cumulative incidence for conventioneers who attended both the luncheon and the dance was 55 percent, with 95 percent confidence bounds of 44 and 65 percent. (In the above calculation, an extra digit has been retained in the values derived in intermediate steps for accuracy. In practice, all intermediate values should be retained with as many digits as possible, with rounding employed only for the final result.)

The calculation of the confidence interval above has two important limitations. First, the method employed is a *large sample* technique, whose accuracy improves as the number of study subjects becomes larger. When the smallest count involved in the calculation is larger than 30, then the results are virtually identical to more accurate methods of calculation, which can be found in intermediate textbooks of epidemiology or statistics. When the smallest count is ten or greater, the results are close enough for most any purpose; when the smallest count is five or less, the method gives bounds that are only roughly indicative of the range of parameter values.

The second important feature is that the method assumes independence of individual results. The risk in any individual is assumed not to be affected by the outcome in other individuals. In contemporary epidemiology, this means that the method given is inappropriate when the number of ill persons is the result of person-to-person transmission of risk.

The variance of the cumulative incidence difference can be estimated by summing the estimated variances of the cumulative incidences that make up the cumulative incidence difference. (See Chapter 13 for rules about the manipulation of variances.) An estimate of the variance associated with the cumulative incidence difference between the dancers attending the luncheon and those not doing so is

$$\text{Var}(CID) \doteq \frac{47(86-47)}{86^3} + \frac{11(77-11)}{77^3}$$

$$= 0.004472$$

Thus

$$CID = \frac{47}{86} - \frac{11}{77}$$

$$= 0.4037$$

and the 95 percent confidence bounds for the difference in the probabilities of pharyngitis are

$$\text{lower} = 0.4037 - 1.96\sqrt{0.004472}$$

$$= 0.273$$

$$\text{upper} = 0.4037 + 1.96\sqrt{0.004472}$$

$$= 0.535$$

*Summarizing experience across several strata.* The cumulative incidence differences associated with attending the luncheon in those who attended the dance and in those who did not attend the dance are somewhat different (40.4 percent and 32.3 percent, respectively). There are a variety of ways in which these two estimates might be summarized in a single overall figure. One approach is to take a weighted average of dancers' and nondancers' cumulative incidences among the luncheon attendees, and then to do the same for the nonattendees, using the same weights. The weighted averages are said to be *adjusted* for the effects of attendance at the dance. Because the same weighting scheme is used to adjust the rates of the luncheon "exposed" and "unexposed" groups, the comparison between exposure groups is a valid one. The resulting weighted averages are referred to as *standardized* cumulative incidences.

**Standardization.** *Standardized measures are formed from a series of individual measures by taking a weighted average of the individual values.*

**Standard.** *The set of weights used for standardization is the standard. These weights sum to 1.*

One convenient standard is the distribution of dancers among luncheon attendees. Of the attendees, 86/(86+23) or 78.9 percent went to the dance, and 23/(86+23), or 21.1 percent, did not. Call the cumulative incidences that are standardized over categories of dance attendance the *standardized cumulative incidences (SCI)*. The cumulative incidences for dancers and nondancers among luncheon attendees were 47/86 (54.7 percent) and 8/23 (34.8 percent), respectively. The *SCI* for luncheon attendees is

$$SCI\,(\text{exposed}) = \left(\frac{86}{86+23}\right)\left(\frac{47}{86}\right) + \left(\frac{23}{86+23}\right)\left(\frac{8}{23}\right)$$

$$= 0.5046$$

For those who did not attend the luncheon, the cumulative incidences among dancers and nondancers were 11/77 (14.3 percent) and 1/40 (2.5 percent), respectively. The *SCI* for nonattendees is

$$SCI\,(\text{unexposed}) = \left(\frac{86}{86+23}\right)\left(\frac{11}{77}\right) + \left(\frac{23}{86+23}\right)\left(\frac{1}{40}\right)$$

$$= 0.1180$$

The standardized cumulative incidence difference (*SCID*) is the difference between the standardized cumulative incidences.

$$SCID = SCI\,(\text{exposed}) - SCI\,(\text{unexposed})$$

$$= 0.3866$$

Note that this result is identical to the result that would be obtained by applying the standard weights to the stratum-specific cumulative incidence differences. The cumulative incidence differences are 0.4037 for those who attended the dance and (8/23)-(1/40) = 0.3228 for those who did not. Standardized over categories of dance attendance, the cumulative incidence difference would be

$$SCID = \left(\frac{86}{86+23}\right)(0.4037) + \left(\frac{23}{86+23}\right)(0.3228)$$

$$= 0.3866$$

The standardized cumulative incidence difference can be seen as a weighted average of the component cumulative incidence differences.

The variance of a weighted average is given by the sum of the component variances, each weighted by the square of the corresponding weight, so that

$$Var(SCID) = \left(\frac{86}{86+23}\right)^2 (0.004472)$$

$$+ \left(\frac{23}{86+23}\right)^2 (0.01047)$$

$$= 0.003250$$

95 percent confidence bounds to the SCID are therefore

$$lower = 0.3866 - 1.96\sqrt{0.003250}$$

$$= 0.2749$$

$$upper = 0.3866 + 1.96\sqrt{0.003250}$$

$$= 0.4983$$

The luncheon "effect" is standardized according to the dancing choices of those who actually attended the lunch. The final measure is intuitively satisfying in that it is directly tied to the experience of the exposed group: it addresses the question "What would have been the difference between those who attended the luncheon and those who did not if the nonattendees had the same fraction of dancers as those who attended?" Other weighting schemes that might have been used include an external standard (such as equal weights for each group), or an internal standard based on the reciprocals of the variances[57] of the stratum-specific cumulative incidence differences. This last standard minimizes the variance of the final

---

57. The reciprocal of the variance of an estimate is also known as the "information" contained in the estimate. Very precise estimates have small variance and high information.

estimate, but its proper use presupposes that the only source of discrepancy between the stratum-specific cumulative incidence differences is chance.

*Confounding.* If the interest in Table 5.1 had focussed on the cumulative incidence difference associated with attendance at the dance, the investigators could have calculated estimates of (47/86) - (8/23) or 20 percent in those who attended the luncheon and (11/77) - (1/40) or 12 percent in those who did not. Any standardized estimate of an overall effect would lie between these two values. If luncheon attendance were ignored, a crude cumulative incidence difference might also have been calculated as

$$CID = \frac{47+11}{86+77} - \frac{8+1}{23+40}$$

$$= 0.213$$

or 21 percent. This value lies outside of the range of stratum-specific estimates. Because luncheon attendance was more common among dancers than among those who did not dance, the crude cumulative incidence difference reflects a part of the cumulative incidence associated with luncheon attendance, in addition to the effect of dance attendance on risk. The crude cumulative incidence difference therefore provides a biased estimate of the increase in probability of pharyngitis associated with attendance at the dance.

**Analysis of Open Cohort Studies**

Example 5.2 will be used to illustrate the techniques presented here.

*Error estimates and comparisons of incidence rates.* Just as the observed proportion of the disease in a closed cohort study is an estimate of the underlying probability of developing disease, so the ratio of cases to person time, the incidence rate, provides an estimate of the underlying hazard of disease. The most straightforward technique for assessing the variability of incidence rates in open cohort studies is based on a treatment of the incidence rate calculation as if the numerator (the number of cases) were variable and the denominator (the amount of person time) were fixed. If $x$ is the number of observed events and $P$ is the person time at risk, then $x$ is the realization of what is called a Poisson process. The probability distribution from which $x$ is drawn is the Poisson distribution.[58]

**Poisson distribution** *is the probability distribution that describes the number of events observed in a block of person time when the expected number of events is directly proportional to the total person time of observation. Let $\theta$ be the expected number of events per unit of person time and $\lambda = \theta P$ be the number of events expected in a block of person time of size $P$.*

$$\Pr(x) = \frac{\lambda^x e^{-\lambda}}{x!}$$

$$E(X) = \lambda$$

$$\mathrm{Var}(X) = \lambda$$

*The range of possible values for $x$ is $[0, \infty)$. $\lambda$ is the Poisson parameter. If $P$ is imagined as being composed of a very large number of discrete units of person time, so that the probability of an event in any person time unit is very small, then the probability distribution of the number of events in $P$ may also be considered to be binomial, with $N$ taken as the number of discrete person time units. All the formulas above are derivable from their binomial counterparts in the limiting case in which $N$ approaches infinity, with $P$ and $\lambda$ constant.*

The number of observed events $x$ is an estimate of a Poisson parameter $\lambda$. The incidence rate estimate $IR$ is given by $x/P$, with variance $x/P^2$.[59] The mortality rate estimate and its variance for the period from 30 through 34 years since first exposure (Table 5.2) are given by

---

58. The development here presumes that the expected number of cases is directly proportional to the amount of person time of observation. Put another way, we presume that there is no element of contagion, in which the probability of a case occurring is a function of the number of other cases that have occurred.

59. c.f. Table 1.2 and Chapter 13. Note that

$$IR = \frac{x}{P}$$

$$\frac{IR}{P} = \frac{x}{P^2}$$

$$IR = \frac{103}{11,598}$$

$$= 0.008881 \text{ cases per person year}$$

$$\mathrm{Var}(IR) = \frac{103}{(11,598)^2}$$

$$= 7.657 \times 10^{-7}$$

The 95 percent confidence bounds are

$$\mathrm{lower} = 0.00881 - 1.96\sqrt{7.657 \times 10^{-7}}$$

$$= 0.00717 \text{ cases per person year}$$

$$\mathrm{upper} = 0.00881 + 1.96\sqrt{7.657 \times 10^{-7}}$$

$$= 0.01060 \text{ cases per person year}$$

All the techniques for estimating incidence rate differences and summary incidence rate changes over strata are precisely analogous to those presented earlier for risks in closed cohort studies. The sole differences are to introduce incidence rate estimates $(x/P)$ in the place of cumulative incidence estimates $(x/N)$ and variance estimates for incidence rates $(x/P^2)$ in the place of variance estimates for cumulative incidences $(x(N-x)/N^3)$ in all the formulae.

It is common practice to examine the ratios of incidence rates in open cohort studies; this is the result of an empirical observation in chronic disease research, that incidence rate ratios tend to be more constant from study to study or from stratum to stratum of a single study than are rate differences. The easiest way to account for variability in incidence ratio estimates is on a logarithmic scale, in which the ratio estimate can be examined as a difference between the logarithms of the component incidence rate estimates. All of the foregoing procedures can then be adapted to confidence interval estimation on the log scale. Estimates, once obtained, are transformed back to the natural scale by exponentiation.

Denote the natural logarithm of the incidence rate estimate as $\ln(x/P)$. The variance of this quantity is approximately $1/x$. The variance of the logarithm of the incidence rate ratio is the sum of the variances of the logarithms of the component incidence rates.

Thus, to compare the lung cancer rate at 30-34 years after first exposure to that 20-24 years after first exposure, the procedure would be as follows:

$$RR = \left(\frac{103}{11,598}\right) / \left(\frac{57}{31,268}\right)$$

$$= 4.87$$

$$\ln(RR) = \ln(4.87)$$

$$= 1.5834$$

$$\text{Var}[\ln(RR)] = \frac{1}{103} + \frac{1}{57}$$

$$= 0.02725$$

The 95 percent confidence bounds for the logarithm of the ratio are

$$\text{lower} = 1.5834 - 1.96\sqrt{0.02725}$$

$$= 1.260$$

$$\text{upper} = 1.5834 + 1.96\sqrt{0.02725}$$

$$= 1.907$$

The 95 percent confidence bounds for the ratio are then

$$\text{lower} = \exp(1.260)$$

$$= 3.52$$

$$\text{upper} = \exp(1.907)$$

$$= 6.73$$

The ratio of lung cancer mortality rates for insulation workers 30-34 years from first exposure to asbestos to that 20-24 years from first exposure was approximately 4.9, with 95 percent confidence bounds of 3.5 and 6.7.

*Stratified analysis.* Two techniques are commonly used for summarizing incidence rate ratios across strata. Consider the hypothetical data in Table 8.1. The first subscript on the symbols displayed indicates the presence (1) or absence (0) of exposure, and the second subscript indicates the age group: 50-54 (1) or 55-59 (2).

**Table 8.1** Lung cancer mortality in men exposed and unexposed to asbestos (hypothetical data)

|  | Age Group | | | |
|  | 50 - 54 | | 55 - 59 | |
|  | Quantity | Symbol | Quantity | Symbol |
|---|---|---|---|---|
| *Exposed* | | | | |
| Person Years | 1,000 | $P_{11}$ | 500 | $P_{12}$ |
| Cases | 40 | $x_{11}$ | 40 | $x_{12}$ |
| *Unexposed* | | | | |
| Person Years | 10,000 | $P_{01}$ | 15,000 | $P_{02}$ |
| Cases | 100 | $x_{01}$ | 200 | $x_{02}$ |

The summary technique most used in occupational health studies is to compare the number of cases of disease in the exposed group to that which would have been expected among the exposed, had the incidence rates observed in unexposed persons applied to those exposed. This expectation is obtained by multiplying the person years at risk in each stratum of the exposed group by the incidence rates observed in the unexposed group, and summing over all strata. Thus, in exposed workers,

$$\text{Observed} = x_{11} + x_{12}$$

$$= 40 + 40$$

$$= 80$$

$$\text{Expected} = P_{11}\frac{x_{01}}{P_{01}} + P_{12}\frac{x_{02}}{P_{02}}$$

$$= 1,000\left(\frac{100}{10,000}\right) + 500\left(\frac{200}{15,000}\right)$$

$$= 16.67$$

The ratio of observed to expected cases is designated (for historical reasons) as "the" *standardized mortality (or morbidity) ratio* (*SMR*). The ratio is standardized because it is algebraically identical to the ratio of age-standardized incidence rates in exposed and unexposed study subjects, taking for each the age distribution among exposed as the standard. In the present case

$$SMR = \frac{Obs}{Exp} = \frac{80}{16.67}$$

$$= 4.80$$

In practice, the $SMR$ is rarely used except when the unexposed population is very large (most commonly a geographically defined population that encompasses the exposed persons). When the number of events is large in every stratum of the comparison population, the variance of the $SMR$ is approximately $Obs/Exp^2$. In the present example

$$Var(SMR) = \frac{Obs}{Exp^2} = \frac{80}{(16.67)^2}$$

$$= 0.2880$$

The 95 percent confidence bounds can be obtained therefore as

$$lower = 4.800 - 1.96\sqrt{0.2880}$$

$$= 3.75$$

$$lower = 4.800 + 1.96\sqrt{0.2880}$$

$$= 5.85$$

When the sole source of stratum to stratum variation is thought to be random error, an incidence rate ratio estimate whose form is due to Mantel and Haenszel[60] is obtainable by summing the quantities

$$A_i = \frac{x_{1i}P_{0i}}{P_{1i} + P_{0i}} \qquad\qquad B_i = \frac{x_{0i}P_{1i}}{P_{1i} + P_{0i}}$$

over the strata, indexed here by $i$, and dividing the sums. In the present example,

60. The use of the procedure in open cohort studies was first proposed by Kenneth Rothman and John Boice. (Rothman KJ, Boice JR. Epidemiologic Analysis with a Programmable Calculator, NIH Publication No. 79-1649, Washington, 1979) The rationale was developed by David Clayton. (Clayton DG. The analysis of prospective studies of disease etiology. Commun Statist 1982;A11:2129-2155)

$$A = \sum_i A_i = \frac{(40)(10,000)}{10,000+1,000} + \frac{(40)(15,000)}{15,000+500}$$

$$= 75.07$$

$$B = \sum_i B_i = \frac{(100)(1,000)}{10,000+1,000} + \frac{(200)(500)}{15,000+500}$$

$$= 15.54$$

(When a variable, here $i$, appears below a sigma without any indication of the range of summation, the summation is taken over all possible values of the variable. In the present example, the possible values for $i$ are 1 and 2.) The summary estimate, known as the *Mantel-Haenszel* estimate of the ratio is

$$RR_{MH} = \frac{A}{B}$$

$$= 4.831$$

The variance of the logarithm of the Mantel-Haenszel estimator is obtained by taking a further sum,

$$C = \sum_i (x_{1i} + x_{0i}) P_{1i} P_{0i} / (P_{1i} + P_{0i})^2$$

The variance estimate is then[61]

$$\text{Var}[\ln(RR_{MH})] \doteq \frac{C}{AB}$$

Here,

$$C = (40+100)(1,000)(10,000)/(1,000+10,000)^2$$

$$+ (40+200)(500)(15,000)/(500+15,000)^2$$

$$= 19.06$$

and

$$\text{Var}[\ln(RR_{MH})] \doteq \frac{19.06}{(75.07)(15.54)} = 0.01634$$

---

61. Greenland S, Robins JM. Estimation of a common effect parameter from sparse follow-up data. Biometrics 1985;41:55–68

The natural logarithm of the hazard ratio estimate is ln(4.831) = 1.575. Proceeding as before, the 95 percent confidence interval to the logarithm of the incidence rate ratio can be found to be 1.325 to 1.826, yielding a corresponding interval on the ratio scale of 3.8 to 6.2.

When the ratios observed in the strata being summarized are not very disparate, when the amounts of person time under study in each exposure group do not vary greatly across strata, or when the person time of the unexposed group is vastly larger than that of the exposed in each stratum, the *SMR* and the Mantel-Haenszel estimate of the incidence rate ratio will be very close to one another, and there is little practical distinction to be made between the two. In the last situation, the closeness of the Mantel-Haenszel estimator to the SMR arises from the fact that both procedures give weight in approximate proportion to the information contained in the exposed half of each stratum.[62] The theory underlying their respective derivations leads to a choice of the *SMR* whenever the stratum-specific hazard ratios are inconstant, and to the Mantel-Haenszel estimator when they do not vary greatly.

## Case-Control Studies

*Random Error.* Analysis of the variability of odds ratios and of more complex functions involving odds ratios is almost always carried out on a logarithmic scale. Expressed as a logarithm, the odds ratio has a simple additive structure:

$$\ln(RR) = \ln\left(\frac{x_1 y_0}{y_1 x_0}\right)$$

$$= \ln(x_1) + \ln(y_0) - \ln(y_1) - \ln(x_0)$$

Here as before "ln($x$)" stands for the natural logarithm of $x$.

An estimate of the variance of the logarithm of a count is given by[63]

62. Walker AM. Small sample properties of some estimators of a common hazard ratio. Appl Statistics 1985;34:42-8

63. The capital X in the formula is the random variable, of which the value x is the observed value.

$$Var[\ln(X)] \doteq \frac{1}{x}$$

Let $O$ stand for the parameter of which the odds ratio is an estimate. Since the variance of the sum or difference of terms equals the sum of the variances of the terms, we have an estimate of the variance of the logarithm of an odds ratio.

$$Var[\ln(O)] = Var[\ln(X_1)] + Var[\ln(X_0)]$$
$$+ Var[\ln(Y_1)] + Var[\ln(Y_0)]$$
$$\doteq \frac{1}{x_1} + \frac{1}{x_0} + \frac{1}{y_1} + \frac{1}{y_0}$$

Approximate 95 percent confidence limits on the log scale are derived by subtracting 1.96 standard errors from $\ln(RR)$ to derive the lower limit, and adding $(1.96 \cdot SE)$ to $\ln(RR)$ to derive the upper limit. Finally, the confidence interval is expressed on the untransformed scale of the $RR$ by exponentiating the limits just obtained.

Using the data from Example 6.1, the variance of the logarithm of the rate ratio is

$$Var[\ln(RR)] = \frac{1}{17} + \frac{1}{2} + \frac{1}{579} + \frac{1}{600}$$
$$= 0.5622$$

The 95 percent confidence interval is

$$lower = \exp[\ln(8.808) - 1.96\sqrt{0.5622}]$$
$$= 2.026$$
$$upper = \exp[\ln(8.808) + 1.96\sqrt{0.5622}]$$
$$= 38.30$$

To two significant digits, the rate ratio is 8.8 with a 95 percent confidence interval of 2.0 to 38.

The dominant term in the variance estimate given above is due to the two controls with a history of undescended testis. Their contribution to the total estimated variance is so great that despite a relatively large number of exposed cases, the overall estimate of effect remains very uncertain, as evidenced by the wide confidence interval. This example illustrates one of the limitations of case-control research: when the exposure under study is rare, estimates are likely to be highly unstable.

*Analysis of Stratified Data.* The most widely used estimate of a summary odds ratio over strata in a case-control study is that of Mantel and Haenszel.[64] The Mantel-Haenszel estimator provides a central value for the odds ratio to which each of the stratum-specific estimates contributes in approximate proportion to its own precision. It is calculated as follows. For each stratum $i$ define the values $x_{1i}$, $x_{0i}$, $y_{1i}$, and $y_{0i}$, as above, and calculate their sum, $T_i$.

$$T_i = x_{1i} + x_{0i} + y_{1i} + y_{0i}$$

Now calculate two more derived quantities for each stratum, $A_i$ and $B_i$.

$$A_i = \frac{x_{1i} y_{0i}}{T_i}$$

$$B_i = \frac{y_{1i} x_{0i}}{T_i}$$

Sum the values of $A$ and $B$ over the strata.

$$A = \sum_i A_i$$

$$B = \sum_i B_i$$

The Mantel-Haenszel summary estimate of the relative rate of disease over strata is

$$RR_{MH} = \frac{A}{B}$$

The parameter estimated by $RR_{MH}$ is a postulated odds ratio that is common to all the strata. Under proper study design, this parameter is identical to the hazard ratio in the source population giving rise to cases and controls. As in the analysis of a single stratum, a confidence interval for the hazard ratio is best calculated on the

64. Mantel N, Haenszel W. Statistical aspects of the analysis of data from retrospective studies of disease. J Natl Cancer Inst 1959;22:719-48

logarithmic scale and then transformed back to the natural scale by exponentiation. In order to obtain an estimate of the variance of the estimator $\ln(RR_{MH})$, it is necessary to calculate several further quantities for each stratum.[65]

$$C_i = \frac{x_{1i} + y_{0i}}{T_i}$$

$$D_i = \frac{y_{1i} + x_{0i}}{T_i}$$

The four derived quantities are combined and summed, stratum by stratum, as follows:

$$(AC) = \sum_i A_i C_i$$

$$(AD) = \sum_i A_i D_i$$

$$(BC) = \sum_i B_i C_i$$

$$(BD) = \sum_i B_i D_i$$

The variance of $\ln(RR_{MH})$ is, approximately,

$$\mathrm{Var}[\ln(RR_{MH})] \doteq \frac{1}{2}\left[\frac{(AC)}{A^2} + \frac{(AD)+(BC)}{AB} + \frac{(BD)}{B^2}\right]$$

As before, the standard error is calculated as the square root of the variance, and 95 percent confidence intervals are obtained on the logarithmic scale by adding and subtracting 1.96 times the standard error to $\ln(RR_{MH})$, after which all of these are transformed back to the original rate ratio scale.

At first glance, the calculation of the 95 percent confidence interval seems a burdensome job, and it does entail a good deal of arithmetic when carried out by hand. An important feature of the formulas is that the data from each stratum need to be processed only once and added to the various accumulating terms. Repeated stratum-by-stratum accumulations are readily accommodated in

65. Robins J, Greenland S, Breslow NE. A general estimator for the variance of the Mantel-Haenszel odds ratio. Am J Epidemiol 1986;124:719-23

spreadsheet programs and programmable calculators. When there is only one stratum, all the above formulas simplify to those given previously for the unstratified case.

**Example 8.1.** *Body mass index and the relative incidence of breast cancer.*[66]

Seventy-two premenopausal women with breast cancer newly diagnosed at the Group Health Cooperative of Puget Sound from July 1975 through June 1978 were interviewed, along with 80 premenopausal women from the same HMO who were hospitalized with a variety of acute conditions. For each subject, the body mass index was ascertained. Women with a body mass index (weight in kilograms divided by the square of height in meters) greater than 28 were classified as "heavy." The first two panels on the left side of Table 8.2 give the distribution of study subjects over categories of disease status, age, and body mass index, together with the age-specific estimates of the rate ratio and the 95 percent confidence intervals.

Calculated values for each of the quantities necessary for the summary estimate of the rate ratio and for the corresponding 95 percent confidence intervals are shown in the right hand panels of Table 8.2, and the resulting estimates are shown in the lower left. Heavy women appear to be at lower risk of breast cancer in both age groups than are other women. Both age-specific estimates are very unstable, because of the small number of heavy women in the study, and particularly so because of the paucity of heavy cases. The common estimate, which accumulates the information available from both strata, is more precise than either of the component values. Note that the common estimate lies within the range of the stratum-specific estimates, as will always be the case.

66. Jick H, Walker AM, Watkins RN, D'Ewart D, et al. Oral contraceptives and breast cancer. Am J Epidemiol 1980;112:577-85

**Table 8.2** Body mass index and the relative incidence of breast cancer among premenopausal women *Calculation of table-specific and summary measures for a case-control study*

| Age $\leq 45$ | | Not | | |
|---|---|---|---|---|
| | Heavy | Heavy | $T_1 = 78$ | |
| | | | $A_1 = 0.7692$ | $A_1C_1 = 0.3156$ |
| Breast Ca | 2 | 35 | $B_1 = 0.4103$ | $A_1D_1 = 0.4536$ |
| | | | $C_1 = 4.9359$ | $B_1C_1 = 2.0250$ |
| Controls | 11 | 30 | $D_1 = 0.5897$ | $B_1D_1 = 2.9109$ |

$$RR = 0.16$$
$$95\% \text{ CI} = 0.032 - 0.76$$

Variance of $\ln(RR) = 0.6528$

| Age $> 45$ | | Not | | |
|---|---|---|---|---|
| | Heavy | Heavy | $T_2 = 73$ | |
| | | | $A_2 = 0.8767$ | $A_2C_2 = 0.4083$ |
| Breast Ca | 2 | 33 | $B_2 = 2.7123$ | $A_2D_2 = 0.4684$ |
| | | | $C_2 = 0.4658$ | $B_2C_2 = 1.2633$ |
| Controls | 6 | 32 | $D_2 = 0.5342$ | $B_2D_2 = 1.4491$ |

$$RR = 0.32$$
$$95\% \text{ CI} = 0.061 - 1.7$$

Variance of $\ln(RR) = 0.7282$

| Summary | | | |
|---|---|---|---|
| | | $A = 1.6459$ | $AC = 0.7239$ |
| | | $B = 7.6482$ | $AD = 0.9220$ |
| $RR_{MH} = 0.22$ | | | $BC = 3.2883$ |
| $95\% \text{ CI} = 0.069 - 0.67$ | | | $BD = 4.3600$ |

Variance of $\ln(RR) = 0.3381$

# 9

# Confounding

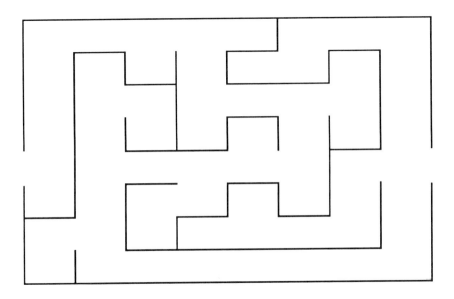

Confounding results from a mixture of effects in a single estimate. An uneven distribution of baseline risks across comparison groups results in a confounded estimate of the differences between the groups. The stratified analyses that were introduced in the last chapter to deal with confounding assumed that the information necessary for segregating study subjects into strata would be available, and a similar requirement holds for mathematical modeling techniques. Often the crucial data are absent. This chapter addresses the strength of bias introduced by confounding when confounding factors are ignored. The approach is entirely theoretical; readers with low tolerance for the abstract may wish to pass directly to the section on Implications at the end.

## The Apparent Relative Risk

Let $E$ stand for an exposure that is either present or absent, and let $Pr(E)$ be the prevalence of one level of $E$ ("exposed") in a population. Let $C$ stand for a covariate characteristic or exposure, also with only two levels, and $Pr(C)$ be the prevalence of one level of $C$ ("possessing the covariate") in the same population. The population prevalences $e$, $f$, $g$, and $h$ displayed in Table 9.1 describe the joint distribution of the population over $E$ and $C$.

**Table 9.1** Prevalences of exposure and covariate

| Covariate | Exposure Present | Absent | Total |
|---|---|---|---|
| Present | $e$ | $f$ | $Pr(C)$ |
| Absent | $g$ | $h$ | $1-Pr(C)$ |
| Total | $Pr(E)$ | $1-Pr(E)$ | $1$ |

Let the population described in Table 9.1 be observed without loss to follow-up for sufficient time to allow the appearance of disease. Assume that the probability of disease is unrelated to exposure, but is a function of covariate status. For population subgroups in which the covariate is present or absent, assume that the probabilities of disease acquisition are $R_c$ or $R_{\bar{c}}$, respectively.

A development exactly analogous to the one that follows can be laid out for cumulative incidences, incidence rates, or hazards, any of which could therefore be substituted for the word "probability" below.

The total probability of disease in exposed persons is

$$R_E = \frac{R_c e + R_{\bar{c}} g}{e + g}$$

That in persons not exposed is

$$R_{\bar{E}} = \frac{R_c f + R_{\bar{c}} h}{f + h}$$

The apparent relative risk, comparing exposed to unexposed segments of the population is

Apparent $RR(E) =$

$$\frac{R_E}{R_{\bar{E}}} = \frac{R_c e + R_{\bar{c}} g}{R_c f + R_{\bar{c}} h} \quad \frac{1 - Pr(E)}{Pr(E)} \qquad [1]$$

Since exposure by definition is not associated with any excess probability of disease, the apparent relative risk is a direct measure of confounding. The first term in the expression above is the exposure odds in cases, the second is the reciprocal of exposure odds in the study population. Since the exposure odds in the control series of a case-control study is a consistent estimate of that in the population in which the cases occurred, the arguments developed here apply to case-control studies as well as to cohort studies.

Define the relative risk comparing persons in whom the covariate is present to those in whom it is absent as

$$RR(C) = \frac{R_c}{R_{\bar{c}}}$$

For fixed overall prevalences of exposure and covariate in the study population, the quantities $f$, $g$, and $h$ can be rewritten as functions of $e$, $Pr(E)$, and $Pr(C)$.

$$f = Pr(C) - e \qquad\qquad g = Pr(E) - e$$
$$h = 1 - Pr(C) - Pr(E) + e$$

On the basis of the preceding expressions, the apparent relative risk for exposure can be rewritten as

Apparent $RR(E) =$

$$\frac{e(RR(C) - 1) + Pr(E)}{(Pr(C) - e)(RR(C) - 1) - Pr(E) + 1} \quad \frac{1 - Pr(E)}{Pr(E)} \qquad [2]$$

The import of Equation 2 is that the degree of confounding introduced into a 2x2 table by the presence of a third, disease-causing factor depends upon the strength of the association between the third factor and disease $(RR(C))$, on the prevalence of exposure $(Pr(E))$, on the prevalence of the third factor $(Pr(C))$, and on the proportion of the study population in which the confounding characteristic and exposure occur together in the same people $(e)$.

Equation 1 can also be written as

Apparent $RR(E) =$

$$\frac{RR(C)e + g}{RR(C)f + h} \quad \frac{1 - Pr(E)}{Pr(E)} \qquad [3]$$

The prevalences of the confounding variable in the exposed and nonexposed segments of the population are

$$Pr(C \mid E) = \frac{e}{Pr(E)} \qquad\qquad Pr(C \mid \overline{E}) = \frac{f}{1 - Pr(E)}$$

Furthermore

$$Pr(\overline{C} \mid E) = \frac{g}{Pr(E)} \qquad\qquad Pr(\overline{C} \mid \overline{E}) = \frac{h}{1 - Pr(E)}$$

By substitution into Equation 3,

Apparent $RR(E) =$

$$\frac{Pr(C \mid E)RR(C) + Pr(\overline{C} \mid E)}{Pr(C \mid \overline{E})RR(C) + Pr(\overline{C} \mid \overline{E})} \qquad [4]$$

**Special Cases and Limits for Apparent RR(E)**

The right hand side of Equation 4 is the ratio of two weighted averages of the quantities $RR(C)$ and 1. (The weights are different, being $P(C \mid E)$ and $P(\overline{C} \mid E)$ in the numerator and $P(C \mid \overline{E})$ and $P(\overline{C} \mid \overline{E})$ in the denominator.) When $RR(C) = 1$, then the Apparent $RR(E) = 1$. When $RR(C) > 1$, the numerator quantity in the ratio is less than $RR(C)$, and the denominator is greater than 1. It follows that

$$\text{Apparent } RR(E) < RR(C) \qquad [5]$$

That the relative risk that could be ascribed to confounding must be less than the relative risk associated with the confounding factor was first observed by Cornfield, Haenszel, and others.[67]

67. Cornfield J, Haenszel W, Hammond EC, Lilienfeld AM, Shimkin MB, Wynder EL. Smoking and lung cancer: Recent evidence and a discussion of some questions. J Nat Cancer Inst 1959;22:173-203 (Appendices A and B)

If $E$ and $C$ are independent, in the sense that

$$e = Pr(E)Pr(C) \qquad [6]$$

then from Equation 2 the Apparent $RR(E)$=1. That is to say, there is no confounding.

From Equation 4 it follows when $RR(C)$>1 and $P(C \mid E) > P(C \mid \bar{E})$ that

$$\text{Apparent } RR(E) < \frac{Pr(C \mid E)}{Pr(C \mid \bar{E})} \qquad [7]$$

I will refer to Equation 7 as "the prevalence inequality." The prevalence inequality holds that the apparent relative risk associated with exposure is less than the ratio of the prevalence of the confounding variable among the exposed to the prevalence of the confounding variable among the nonexposed. When the prevalence of the confounding variable in the study population approaches 100 percent, the degree of confounding approaches nil (Apparent $RR(E)$ = 1). When the prevalence of the confounding variable is zero, the right hand side of Equation 7 is undefined, but it follows from Equation 4 that the Apparent $RR(E)$ = 1 for all values of $RR(C)$ and of $Pr(E)$>0.

Using the notation of Table 9.1, we can write the Exposure-Covariate Odds Ratio ($ECOR$) as

$$ECOR = \frac{eh}{fg}$$

Independence between E and C, in the sense defined by Equation 6, is equivalent to $ECOR$=1. When $ECOR$ is greater than 1, it always exceeds the corresponding ratio of confounder prevalences in the exposed and nonexposed, which in turn exceeds one. That is

$$1 < \frac{Pr(C \mid E)}{Pr(C \mid \bar{E})} < ECOR$$

which in combination with Equation 7 implies that

$$1 < \text{Apparent } RR(E) < ECOR \qquad [8]$$

**Determinants of the Apparent RR(E)**

The results of the preceding section place limits on the degree of confounding that can result from values of *Pr(E)*, *Pr(C)*, *RR(C)*, and the *ECOR*, but they do not provide information on the manner in which the confounding varies as a function of these together. We will approach this question graphically.

Conditionally upon the margins of Table 9.1 and the *ECOR*, *e* can be found as the solution of a quadratic equation. Substitution of the derived value for *e* into Equation 2 yields an expression relating *RR(E)* to *ECOR*, *Pr(C)*, *Pr(E)*, and *RR(C)*. The dependence of the Apparent *RR(E)* on these terms is graphed in Figures 9.1 - 9.3.

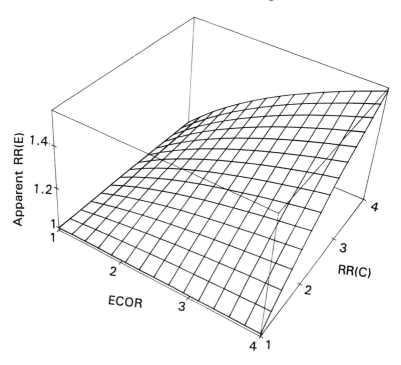

**Figure 9.1** Dependence of the apparent relative risk associated with exposure on the relative risk associated with the covariate and on the exposure-covariate odds-ratio for *Pr(E)*=0.2 and *Pr(C)*=0.2

Figure 9.1 displays the Apparent $RR(E)$ as a function of $RR(C)$ and the $ECOR$ for $Pr(E)=Pr(C)=0.2$. $ECOR$ and $RR(C)$ both range in the figure from 1 to 4. Where $ECOR=RR(C)=1$, the Apparent $RR(E)=1$. So long as $ECOR$ equals unity, the Apparent $RR(E)$ remains unity. The same holds true so long as $RR(C)$ equals unity. For values of $ECOR$ and $RR(C)$ greater than their respective baselines, the Apparent $RR(E)$ rises with increasing association of exposure and covariate and does so with increasing slope as $RR(C)$ increases. Not shown in the figure is the situation when either $ECOR$ or $RR(C)$ falls below one. Then the confounding is in a negative direction, so that the Apparent $RR(E)$ is less than one. When both $ECOR$ and $RR(C)$ are less than one, the confounding is again positive.

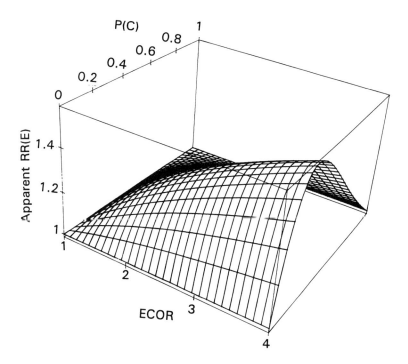

**Figure 9.2** Dependence of the apparent relative risk associated with exposure on the overall prevalence of the covariate and on the exposure-covariate odds-ratio for $Pr(E)=0.2$ and $RR(C)=4$

Figure 9.2 presents the surface described by *Pr(C)*, *ECOR*, and
*RR(E)* for *Pr(E)*=0.2 and *RR(C)*=4. The values of *Pr(C)* in Figure
9.2 range from 0 to 1, and those of the *ECOR* from 1 to 4. Here as
in Figure 9.1, the Apparent *RR(E)* equals one when there is no
association between *E* and *C*, that is, when *ECOR*=1. For larger
values of *ECOR*, the degree of confounding (as measured by the
distance between *RR(E)* and its null value of unity) rises from none
when *Pr(C)*=0 to a maximum (at *Pr(C)*=0.2) and then falls back to
none at *Pr(C)*=1. For values of *ECOR* less than one (not shown in
Figure 9.2), the Apparent *RR(E)* falls below unity, the more so as
*ECOR* approaches 0.

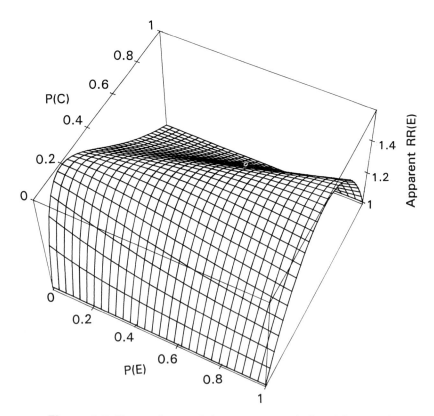

**Figure 9.3** Dependence of the apparent relative risk associated
with exposure on the overall prevalences of exposure and
covariate for *ECOR*=4 and *RR(C)*=4

The relation between the prevalence inequality and Figure 9.2 can be seen most clearly at the upper limit values for $Pr(C)$. When the prevalence of the confounding variable approaches 1, then the ratio of confounding variable prevalence in exposed to that in nonexposed persons must also approach 1, and the Apparent $RR(E)$ approaches 1 as well. As $Pr(C)$ nears zero, the confounding effect approaches the null in what appears to be a smooth manner. At $ECOR=4$, the prevalence of the covariate characteristic that results in the greatest distortion of the apparent relative risk associated with exposure is 0.2.

Figure 9.3 presents the dependence of the Apparent $RR(E)$ on $Pr(E)$ and $Pr(C)$ for the case of $ECOR=5$ and $RR(C)=4$. This figure comprises an expansion of the foremost slice of Figure 9.2, for which $Pr(E)$ was set equal to 0.2. The prevalence of the covariate characteristic associated with the maximum degree of confounding can be seen to increase as the prevalence of exposure rises. It does so in a linear fashion, increasing from $Pr(C)=0.2$ when $Pr(E)$ is near zero to $Pr(C)=0.5$ when $Pr(E)$ is near one.

**Implications**

The degree of confounding is a joint function of the prevalence of exposure $(Pr(E))$, the prevalence of the covariate $(Pr(C))$, the relative risk for disease associated with the covariate $(RR(C))$, and the exposure-covariate odds ratio $(ECOR)$. None of these terms can be considered in isolation from the others if a quantitative interpretation is the goal. Qualitatively,

1. Confounding increases as the strength of the association between disease and the covariate increases (Figure 9.1), but is always less than the relative risk for disease associated with the covariate (Equation 5).

2. Confounding increases as the strength of the association between exposure and the covariate increases (Figures 9.1 and 9.2) but is always less than the ratio of the prevalence of covariate in the exposed to that in the nonexposed group (Equation 7). Equivalently, confounding is always less than the odds ratio between exposure and the covariate (Equation 8).

3. When the covariate is associated positively with exposure and with probability of disease, then the degree of confounding rises smoothly as the prevalence of the covariate increases from zero, reaches a maximum, and then declines toward nil as the covariate prevalence increases further towards one (Figures 9.2 and 9.3).

# 10

# Reporting Results

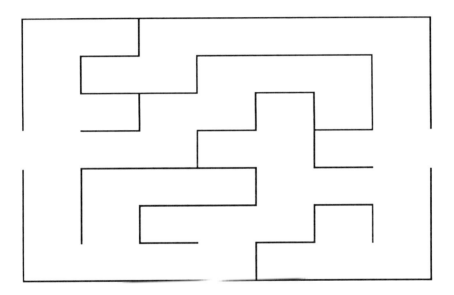

Throughout the conception, design, and analysis of epidemiologic studies, there are points at which anticipating the report that must follow can lead to a more lucid final product. The reader will have to feel in the end that he has been able to disentangle truth from serendipity and bias. He will have to be given sufficient information to judge the quality of the data collection, and the pertinence of those data to the conditions and events that are the real objects of study. He must be guided through a tiny fraction of all the observable relations in the data and yet be convinced that he has grasped the essential information. The purpose of this chapter is to lay out guidelines for communicating results to a reader.

## Context

Begin a report by stating the relations that are to be addressed and the motivations for considering those relations to be of interest. The observations that stimulated the present work may be the product of laboratory efforts, but more often they will stem from case series, correlational studies, or previous formal epidemiologic analyses that suggest an exposure-disease relation. Since the details of exposure and disease definition vary across populations, it may be desirable to do little more than replicate an earlier design. In any case, give the testable implications of other studies as a simply stated, positive hypothesis. Previous findings that are not testable, that is to say refutable, in the work being reported have little relevance.

An important aspect of the study's context, quite different from its scientific antecedents, is its logistical setting. State whether the current work is based on *ad hoc* data collection, is part of a series of studies carried out in the same population, or is an offshoot of a larger study, a multipurpose study, or a surveillance system. Catch phrases to be used later in the text, such as "specially trained interviewers," will take on the coloring of their surroundings, so be sure to offer evidence, even circumstantial, for the extent to which the data emerging from your work can be expected to reflect the reality of the universe under observation. If well-known relations have been reproduced in the data, report as much concisely.

## Study Subjects and the Source Population

Rates, proportions, and functions of these measures underlie all meaningful reports of epidemiologic findings. Each entails the definition of a source population within which the observations are made. The source population may be enumerated, or its definition may be only implicit in the choice of study subjects. In either case it should be described in terms of those features that affect disease frequency and feasibility of data collection. Characteristics that are known prior to initiating the study may be described in the methods section, together with a specification that would permit any given person's inclusion in the source population at any given in time to be determined.

Occasionally an attempt to describe the source population implied by a case selection procedure will highlight an underlying weakness of a study. The source population of cases admitted to a single hospital is a frequently cited example. Several hospitals may serve a single catchment area, and the propensity of patients to choose one or another facility may be related to factors under study, such as ethnic group or income. An investigator's inability to specify his source population in operational terms presages uncertainties throughout design, analysis, and interpretation.

In case-control studies only a sample of the source population (the control series) is actually studied, and its characteristics are taken to represent those of the source population or population time at risk. The sampling mechanism must be described in sufficient detail for the reader to judge whether the selection procedure is likely to have produced a control series that reflects the distribution of characteristics under study in the source population. Response frequencies and characteristics of nonrespondents are of interest. Sometimes control series are chosen in a multistep process that may be only partly under the investigator's control. A diseased control may be "selected" from the source population by his disease, then by the investigator from among all similarly diseased persons, then by himself in agreeing to participate in the study; each step should be examined for possible dependency on exposure status.

However controls are selected, one guiding principle should be evident: within the sampling frame, controls provide unbiased information about the population giving rise to the cases. A helpful way to describe the control series is by presenting the control selection process as homologous to the case selection process: each defines a source population. The two source populations must be identical with respect to determinants of exposure; the simplest practical device to ensure the identity of characteristics is to make the source populations for the two selection processes the same. If the investigator does not have a clear idea as to just which population gives rise to the cases, neither he nor the reader can be expected to judge the adequacy of the controls.

## Data Collection

In describing data sources, provide detail as to who collects and provides the information, how the data are recorded, and the route by which the initial information reaches the form finally analyzed. Note quality control procedures and methods for detecting obviously wrong or inconsistent responses. When the methods used are routine, be brief; when they are novel, be ample (and circumspect). When the detail of the available data puts prior limitations on the questions that can be asked, say so.

**Results**

*Communicate the substance of the data.* There has never been an important epidemiologic observation that could not be clearly presented in a few tables of raw data. Tables of cases and populations at risk or of case and control counts cross-classified by exposure status serve a double purpose of conveying both the substantive message of a set of observations and the uncertainty that may result from small numbers. Often a single 2x2 or 2x$k$ table captures a result, sometimes stratification by an important confounder is needed, seldom is anything more complex required.

Simplicity in data presentation does not mean that analysis should be obtuse. Factors which potentially confound or influence a result must be examined through stratification and appropriate calculation of summary measures, or through statistical modeling. Packages for statistical analysis of epidemiologic data are widely available; multivariate techniques that were once reserved for the last stage of analysis are being used to sift through large numbers of potentially interacting and confounding terms. When this practice is followed responsibly, the analyst's monitoring of changes in parameter estimates, the covariance matrix, and goodness-of-fit measures replace the scanning of tables to get a "feel" for the variability and interrelations in the data.

Whether the analyst's insight derives from the perusal of scores of tables or dozens of regression equations, he has an understanding of the data which cannot be fully communicated under the normal constraints of journal publication; he must accordingly choose the central themes to be presented. While a reader should understand the strategy employed to sort through the data, there is no reason for him precisely to relive the analyst's exploration. An increasingly common and useful practice is to present the simplest tables that capture an effect together with effect estimates based on the most comprehensive feasible analysis.

*Certainty of the estimates.* Confidence intervals provide estimates of a gamut of relations consistent with a given set of observations. They may allow reconciliation of divergent results, and they generally (since confidence intervals are almost always wider than one would wish) introduce an appropriate note of caution into the interpretation of "clear" findings. P values can be useful when no direct estimate of effect is available or readily interpretable, as is sometimes the case with higher order terms in statistical models of rich data sets. For the most part, p values should not be presented in isolation or with a point estimate alone, much less in the degraded form of a statement such as "significant" or "NS." Epidemiologists study and estimate the magnitude of biologic relations, and the dichotomizing effect of an uprooted report of significance is generally out of place.

Neither p values nor confidence intervals provide a full accounting of the uncertainty inherent in the analysis of epidemiologic results. The distinction between observational and experimental data in this respect is that the analyst substitutes a working hypothesis about the nature of unmeasured variables for the physical act of randomization. Both the confidence interval and the p value have simple operational definitions in clinical trials, where the chance mechanism allocates exposure. In an observational study, we hypothesize that measured exposures are distributed as if by chance and we apply techniques proper to the analysis of truly probabilistic phenomena to assess the possible contribution of chance to a study's findings. The proposition that the exposures are distributed in a random fashion, conditionally upon other measured factors, is not testable. Its plausibility should be reviewed in the discussion section of a report under the general heading of uncontrolled confounding.

*Missing data.* Even after subjects have successfully participated in a study, certain items of information may remain missing. Respondents occasionally give uninformative answers to the most carefully posed questions; routine records are commonly incomplete. The frequency with which data are missing for any reason is an important piece of information about the quality of a study and ought to be presented explicitly. A common assumption that permits the simple removal from analyses of subjects with missing data (or occasionally the estimation of what the missing data would have been had they been available) is that the loss of data is a random event, unrelated to the true values of observed quantities. The proposition is sometimes patently false, as when a value is missing because it is out of the range of recordable characteristics, but will more often be subtly wrong as when a crucial variable is censored as a function of a predictor of risk. For example, histological verification of a difficult-to-diagnose tumor may be poor in the very old or unusually accurate in the affluent. In these cases an analysis of the relation between tumor type and any correlate of age or social class will be in error. A minimal safeguard is to present unknowns in every table, and to include "unknown" in multivariate procedures as a distinct category of risk or disease. While serious distortions cannot always be prevented, their presence may be signaled in associations between "unknown" status and disease or risk factors. If unknown responses are common, some consideration of their impact must appear, either in the analysis or in the discussion of results.

*Multiple hypotheses.* Unanticipated results are common when large numbers of factors have been investigated. Within limits imposed by the subjects' ability to provide meaningful responses, the goal of extracting as much information as possible from interviews is worthwhile, but a number of problems present themselves, particularly when the number of cases is not large. The principal difficulties imposed by "too rich" data are multiple comparisons, subgroup analysis, and invalidation of control representativeness. Each of these demands special care in presentation.

The multiple comparisons problem concerns the expectation that tests of a large number of independent hypotheses will lead predictably to statistically significant findings for some of the tests, even under a null hypothesis. When many tests are done at the same time, and when any one of them being statistically significant would constitute an important finding, a frequent recommendation is to decrease the size of the p value required to declare any single finding significant. The extent of the decrease is a function of the number of comparisons being made. Fewer findings are declared significant by the more stringent criterion, but the proposed remedy highlights an unfortunate aspect of dependence on p values, in that it leads to an inability to detect any effect as the required significance level drops toward zero. More serious is that the suggestion often cannot be implemented in any consistent way: the number of independent hypotheses that could be tested in a set of richly interrelated observations may not be determinable from the data at hand, and those hypotheses that might reasonably be tested differ as a function of information external to the study. Should I discount an interesting finding because the investigator tested some hypotheses that I consider absurd? A preferable alternative is to present unanticipated findings and their unadjusted confidence intervals with an appropriate comment identifying the corresponding hypotheses as ones not entertained at the beginning of the study, and to test further implications of the new hypotheses in the data at hand.

The interpretation of unanticipated results depends heavily on external criteria of biologic plausibility and of consistency with other findings. It follows that proper interpretation of a study will change with time; it will continue to evolve long after publication, as new understanding is brought to bear on old data.

Subgroup analysis is a variant of the multiple comparisons problem in which a single hypothesis is multiplied by separate investigation in many subpopulations. Except when strata are few and heavily populated, tests for heterogeneity have low power against many interesting alternatives. Insisting on significant tests of heterogeneity to justify subgroup analysis protects the analyst from being distracted by the inconsequential; the cost is an almost total inability to recognize true variation. Relevant observations external to the study are usually crucial to the decision to take an observed subgroup effect seriously.

Often, control series that are not chosen by random sampling from a well-defined population are tailored to specific studies. Hospital controls might be selected from persons with diagnoses thought not to be associated with alcohol or tobacco consumption in a study that addresses the effects of those exposures. Such a series may provide valid estimates of alcohol and tobacco use, yet highly biased estimates of the prevalence of other habits related to diagnoses used to specify controls. One way to reduce risk of error in this situation is to choose control diagnoses by inclusion (rather than by exclusion) and to present exposure frequencies within control categories. In general, however, it is wise to limit exploratory case-control analyses to studies in which the process that generates controls has a small number of well defined and quantifiable steps. The simplest case holds when classical survey sampling methods generate the controls for population-based cases.

## Implications

The impetus for epidemiologic studies may come from many disciplines, and the implications of an observation may be broad. Nonetheless, it is rare that epidemiologic results themselves justify lengthy mechanistic discussion. The commentary should place the results in the context of relevant work, drawing parallels where possible, and highlighting points of conflict. Findings inconsistent with previous hypotheses are more likely than confirmatory results to lead to new insight, and divergences should be explored with as much care as the data permit.

# 11

# Risk Perception and Communication

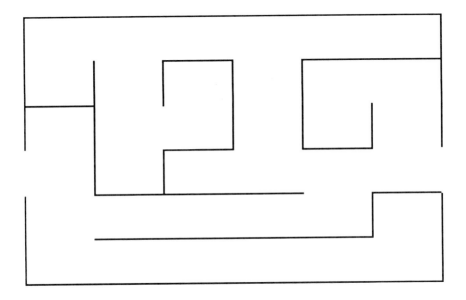

An anomaly of human behavior known to casualty insurers is the "earthquake paradox." Sales of insurance policies rise dramatically following an earthquake, then gradually fall off. By contrast, the risk of another disaster is lowest immediately following a serious temblor, and rises steadily with the passage of time. Even populations in which the time course of the risk is widely known exhibit the paradoxical behavior, which redounds to the insurer's benefit, but leaves the society ill-served. Mathematically irrational behaviors, such as the earthquake paradox, arise when the scale in which a behavior is valued by an individual is not a linear function of expected return.

## Economic Reason and the Quantification of Risk

Statisticians quantify chancy behavior with the idea of the "expected value" of a decision. The expected value is a summation taken over all the possible outcomes of a chance process. In the present case, we consider the chance process that is set in motion by a particular course of action. We might thus talk about the expected value of cardioversion in the treatment of arrhythmia, the expected value of a pollution control law, or the expected value of buying a lottery ticket.

In each case, the same formal logic applies. The value of every possible outcome is assessed in terms of a measurable result: the number of lives or days of life gained or lost, the gains from each degree of remediation of an environmental ill, the cost of a losing lottery ticket, or the value of the jackpot. For each possible outcome, the corresponding value is multiplied by the probability that the outcome will ensue from the decision taken. The products of value times probability, summed over all the possible outcomes, yield the expected value of the decision.

$$E(Value) = \sum_i Value_i f_i$$

where "$Value_i$" is the value of the $i$th outcome, which occurs with probability, or relative frequency, $f_i$.

The procedure is straightforward when the decision is whether to enter into a wager. Place a hundred dollar bet on the black numbers in a game of roulette. The value of the ball's landing on black is a gain of $100, the value of its landing on red is a $100 loss, as is the value of the ball's landing on green. The corresponding probabilities are 18 parts in 38, 18 in 38, and 2 in 38, so that the value of the bet is $100x(18/38) - $100x(18/38) - $100x(2/38) or a loss of $5.26.

A probability is an expected average of real outcomes, forecast into the future. As noted at the beginning of this book, attaching the word probability to a particular event is really a statement of the class to which the event belongs. With a fair roulette wheel, there is no ambiguity in specifying the class to which a single spin belongs, and probabilistic statements accurately characterize the long-run performance of the system.

The economic basis for considering the expected value of a decision is solid when the number of decisions to be made is large. The casino earns money in the gaming example because the long run return on many bets averages out to $5.26 per $100 bet. An insurance policy is akin to a bet. The wager is the premium and the payoff is the avoidance of loss. The expected return on an insurance policy is the sum of the probability of each possible payout multiplied by its value. The difference between the expected returns of many policies (bets) and the total premium (wagers) is the insurer's profit. A lottery ticket analogously has an expected return equal to the size of the jackpot multiplied by the probability of winning, and the difference between the ticket's expected value and the price is the state's average take. The average take has only a highly theoretical meaning on the level of the individual ticket, but the sum over many tickets is a favorite means of state finance.

The expected value of a probabilistic decision has a close connection to the worth that an individual attaches to the decision. The arena in which the relation holds is that within which the individual can experience a sufficient number of repeated times at risk that his total return or loss can be predicted with precision from the sum of expected values. A scofflaw who parks his car in an illegal spot may observe that the expected value of his action is cheaper than paying for a parking lot. If the probability of paying for a parking citation multiplied by the amount of the fine is less than the cost of parking legally for a day, then the choice is economically rational.

When the chance decision involves outcomes that are very rare and either very costly or very advantageous, expected value becomes a poor index of the perceived utility of a decision. Humans place a worth on the possible catastrophe or bonanza that exceeds the expected value. This is the basis of both insurance schemes and lotteries. In Massachusetts, the state with the highest per capita sales of lottery tickets in North America, the public readily accepts a jackpot that is less than 70 percent of the total take.[68] Similarly, and with good reason, I am willing to pay for automobile liability insurance a premium that exceeds the expected value, or the product of the chance of my having a costly accident multiplied by the damages. An excess cost of automobile insurance over and above the expected value of the policy of 20 or 30 percent does not seem

---

68. Branch T. What's wrong with the lottery? New England Monthly 1989;7:40-9

unacceptable to most buyers. In both these instances, note that paying out more than the expected value does not result from lack of information on the part of the insured or the bettor.

The psychology that may underlie decision making in risky situations has been characterized by the "minimax" criterion. The term "minimax" is a shorthand for a strategy that involves "minimizing the maximum foreseeable loss." If I buy catastrophe insurance, I reduce the loss in case of catastrophe to the amount of the insurance premium. The cost in the absence of catastrophe is higher than it would have been had I not purchased insurance, but the expected small loss (paying the premium) is irrelevant to a minimax player. Minimax strategies are appealing when the individual is unlikely to experience all possible outcomes in the course of his risk-taking career. Pascal's wager was an example of minimax: he reasoned that the inconvenience of professing Catholicism was an acceptably small known loss, since it permitted the faithful to avoid the alternative (however unlikely) of perpetual damnation.

Insurance systems and lotteries provide a satisfactory social arrangement because they present a collaboration between two kinds of entities: the individual and the collective. The individual, with little expectation of great loss or major gain, plays the minimax strategy. He pays a surcharge over an expected value that has no direct meaning to him. The collective plays a game of expected value. The casino, the state, the underwriter all anticipate so many wagers that the overall return will approximate the expected value. Both sides win, in a sense, but observe that the system works because the collective interest (in selling the insurance policy or the lottery ticket) is just the opposite of the individual interest.

### The Attribution of Risk

An analysis of expected value depends on the idea that the magnitude of risk is well understood, and can be entered into a mathematical balance.

Although gaming strategies such as minimax may have an intuitive, even genetic, basis that guides daily behavior, risk quantification is a relative newcomer to the intellectual scene.[69] Until the Renaissance, there was no recorded mathematical treatment of

---

69. Hacking, I. The Emergence of Probability. Cambridge University Press. Cambridge 1975

chance, and even then the relation between the long-range behavior of dice and inference about the nature of dice was not evident. The notion of probabilistic evidence that emerged around 1660 drew on two completely separate sources. One had to do with degree of belief. Teachings that enjoyed the approbation of church authorities (teachings that were "probable") were judged more likely to be true than were heretical positions. The second drew on the low sciences of alchemy and medicine. "Signs," empirical correlates of past events, were accepted as having predictive value.

Attribution of the individual to a risk class is based entirely on what would have been called "signs" in the Middle Ages. Signs then and now may be misread, and the resulting misclassification of individuals results in a misattribution of the causes of risk.

The element of risk attribution that follows after classification is the assertion that a proportion of the members of the class will manifest an outcome. The experience of the analysis of dice is particularly apropos: the behavior of fair dice can be approached empirically, in a thousand or ten thousand throws; or it can be investigated theoretically, utilizing the abstract concept of "fair dice" to derive a probability distribution. The sad connection to environmental risk assessment, however, is that neither approach seems to hold promise. The interrelations of environmental toxins with one another and with the environment are sufficiently varied that there is little opportunity to gain repeated or repeatable empirical data on health effects in the field. At the same time, the theoretical approach that comes out of isolated laboratory observation cannot yet begin to address the expected behavior of real systems. For risk assessments based on intense and repeated exposures, such as tobacco smoke, workplace toxins, alcohol, or drugs, the basis for inference is much stronger. In every case, epidemiologists or their critics ought to be alert to define the limits of that which can be reasonably achieved.

## The Perception of Risk

The social and political assessment of risk bears more kinship to the approbation of church fathers than it does to the search for the operational rules of a pair of dice. Most frequently, despite expert assessments, the likely outcomes are only guessed at. Here the psychology of wagers and insurance schemes may still apply, but the choices are predicated on perceived risk.

Try a thought experiment. Imagine yourself in Québec, a city for conventioneers and tourists in a region that has experienced little seismic activity for three centuries. Across the continent there has been a disaster in another attractive city, San Francisco, and seismologists are predicting that "the big one," a devastating earthquake, will occur within the next 30 years with near certainty. Go in your thoughts from Québec to San Francisco for a few days. Most people who seriously engage their imagination in the fantasy can sense the anxiety of change from a region of low risk to one of high risk. The thrill of speeding in a car is similarly related to the transition from a low-risk state (driving slowly or not at all) to a high-risk one.

Residents of New York City, who are accustomed to muggings and street crime, feel immediately safer, they "unwind," when they vacation in the countryside. The change in risk is acutely perceived.

For comparison, now carefully imagine that you move with your family to San Francisco. You experience some trepidation at first. No earthquake occurs for a month, a year, ten years. Can you feel the "earthquake paradox" taking hold? You *are* more comfortable. In the same way the New Yorker adapts to his world. These illustrations suggest that we are more conscious of change-in-risk than we are of absolute levels of danger. Whatever level of risk we find ourselves in for a long period, we adapt to. Whenever the level changes, we are alert.

Many examples of risk seeking or risk aversion seem intuitively obvious to observers brought up in widely different cultures, to such an extent that studies that demonstrate these behaviors could almost be performed as thought experiments. My personal speculation is that the sensitivity to change has a survival value when the change is between levels of risk that are uncertain. New, but unknown, risk levels may be unacceptably high, may be catastrophic, or may require special precautions. If australopithecus scanning the savannah to protect his migrating band is too romanticized an image, consider the Manhattan dandy who drives by mistake into South Bronx: there is a survival value to anxiety in the face of change in risk. A life-preserving choice of action in the face of imperfect risk data would confer a Darwinian advantage comparable to that of the opposing thumb. Put aside for a moment the evidence that evolution involves as much happenstance as direction; we may wonder whether risk-taking behavior, like color vision, the sense of time, or the visual calculus of depth, has not in some way been optimized for safe behavior.

How much change alerts us? Consider your lifetime risk of myocardial infarction. If you are male, aged 40, a nonsmoker, and a vegetarian, your risk may be on the order of 20 percent. If you eat animal products, the risk may be 25 percent or so. Does the difference justify a change in diet? The cost is more modest than moving out of an earthquake zone, the change in risk many orders of magnitude larger in absolute terms, yet very few persons, even among those who accept the data, actually change their habits. Absolute change in risk seems not to be key to behavior change.

Studies of risk perception have included attempts to have people estimate the relative ranking of commonly discussed risks, such as the probability of being struck by lightning, of having an automobile accident, or of developing cancer within the next year. Study subjects can distinguish risks that differ from one another by a factor of ten with some reliability, but risks closer to one another are frequently confused. The relation holds over a wide range of absolute risks. Relative risk, the epidemiologic measure that compares the ratio of risk in one group to risk in another, appears to correspond, largely by accident, to a measure that people can grapple with.

**Implications for Communication**

There are a number of rules for discussing risk that arise from the points presented here:

Perhaps the most important is *do not expect quantitative discussions of risk to carry the day.* Neither the proponent of a decision nor the antagonist has a sufficiently well-developed intuition about the meaning of risk. The issue is not one of training, but rather of the neuropsychology of risk perception.

The next is *accept minimax.* Worst-case scenarios are not a perversion or a rhetorical tool. They are a natural manifestation of the psychology of risk perception. When the risks involved are societal, when an entire population is at risk for a single event, then the expected value rationale may not be justifiable.

*Translate linear decisions into economic terms.* Risk comparisons in personal perception and public debate are inherently nonlinear. If you are working in a situation in which expected value is meaningful, then set an economic meaning for expected value, and discuss that. A 30 percent risk reduction has less appeal than a 30 percent cut in taxes.

Finally recognize that *the rhetoric of risk is subject to manipulation*. Choose your baseline with care, but do not pretend to do so with the object of conveying a uniquely valid truth. Suppose that we believe that a novel chemical exposure causes leukemia in a small fraction of exposed persons. The risk may be smaller than that of cancer from a sunburn, yet still it may be advertised as a hundred times larger than the leukemia risk attributable to all manmade sources of radiation combined; opponents may counter that the same risk is less than a tenth of the risk is that attributable to viral infections, or a thousandth of the lifetime all-cause cancer mortality risk. The "meaning" is what you choose to make of it.

# 12

# Questions for Review

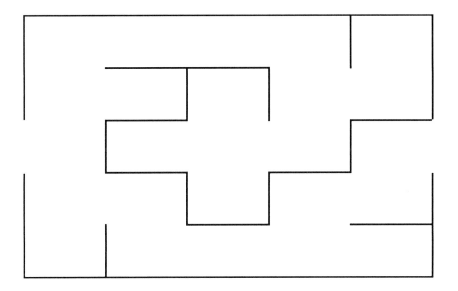

We have very little direct experience of risks or rates in our personal lives, and as a consequence, intuition about the right choices to make in designing a study often fails, even in persons who seem to have a grasp of epidemiologic theory. The questions that follow are intended to retrace the ground covered in such a way as to challenge the reader's grasp of the fundamentals and their implications.

**Disease Frequency**

When the size of the population under observation is one, what values of risk can be observed? What probabilities of disease might characterize the individual who constitutes the observed population?

The prevalence of a characteristic may change within a given population over time. Describe one way in which a population prevalence can change without any member changing with respect to the characteristic, and one in which the population does not change although many of the members change.

Can a person become an incident case of a disease while he has the disease? How does the foregoing answer help define the population that should be studied for an estimate of incidence?

The experience of even a single individual comprises many different periods with different time-bound characteristics. How can the experiences of many individuals be aggregated for study into pools within which there is a homogeneity of characteristics?

If a personal characteristic affects the mean duration of disease in individuals who have acquired the disease, but does not affect the incidence of disease, how will the characteristic affect prevalence?

**Comparisons**

The incidence rate of hepatic adenoma in oral contraceptive users is at least fifty times that in nonusers. Oral contraceptive use is common, yet the population rate difference for hepatic adenoma due to oral contraceptive use is tiny. As a consequence, what must be true of the incidence rate of hepatic adenoma?

The rate of subacute sclerosing panencephalitis (SSPE) in persons who have suffered measles 30 to 59 days previously is on the order of one per 6,000 person months (assume that one person month equals 30 person days), and is approximately zero at other times. Prior to the availability of measles immunization, the prevalence of persons who had measles among urban ten year olds in the United States was approximately 90 percent. In that pre-immunization era, approximately what was the cumulative incidence of SSPE from birth to age 10?

The rate of cataract formation among long-term users of high doses of systemic steroids is approximately five times that in otherwise comparable populations, yet the population rate difference for cataract due to systemic steroid use in the United States is small. What can you conclude about systemic steroid use?

"The incidence of myocardial infarction doubles with every five-year increase in age after age forty in smoking men." Write down a model of incidence that describes this relation, using the following terms: $a$, the age in years; $I_a$, the incidence at age $a$; and $I_{40}$, the incidence at age 40.

### Study Types

Refer to Figure 3.1. Describe one causal hypothesis suggested by the data and suggest the design of a study that might test that hypothesis.

In order to assess the present need for services to residents of Massachusetts with Downs' Syndrome, would you need to conduct a survey, a cohort study, or a case-control study?

Working at the Massachusetts Cancer Registry, you notice a number of cases of Down's syndrome among newly diagnosed cases of acute lymphocytic leukemia of childhood. Assume that all cases of leukemia are notified to the Cancer Registry and that you can readily determine whether any notified case is also someone with Down's syndrome. How might you integrate the results of the previous study (given in the answer to the question above) with the Cancer Registry data in order to estimate the relative rate of leukemia as a function of the presence of Down's syndrome? What kind of study have you done?

Phenylpropanolamine (PPA) is a common over-the-counter decongestant, used by people with upper respiratory infections. You wish to examine the possibility that use of PPA increases the incidence of stroke within 24 hours of use. Describe the study subjects, the exposure and outcome data, and the comparisons that would be required for each of the following studies of this question: a closed cohort study, an open cohort study, a case-control study.

**Time**

Caffeine affects myocardial irritability for six hours following consumption of a cup of coffee. Would lifetime coffee consumption be a helpful measure of caffeine exposure for a study of the risk of disease events that are determined by myocardial irritability?

After infection with HIV, a period ensues during which the virus multiplies and progressively destroys immunocompetent cells. Early in this period, there is no alteration in any aspect of the victim's immunocompetence. Of what time-related phenomenon is the interval from infection to first symptom an example? If you were studying the effects of HIV, how would you interpret the person time and any disease events that accrue in this interval?

The incidence of adult onset asthma rises abruptly for workers who enter an occupational setting that requires contact with allergenic agents. The incidence then declines with progressive time since entry into the setting. Offer possible explanations for the decline that invoke the distinction between inception and survivor cohorts.

Are the results displayed in Figures 3.4 and 3.5 examples of period effects or cohort effects?

**Cohort Studies**

Refer to Example 5.1. In the context of that study, was a conventioneer who attended the luncheon but did not eat the chicken salad and was not exposed to group G streptococcus a member of a population "at risk"? Was a conventioneer who ate the chicken salad but did not furnish any information about his activities a member of a population at risk?

Some commentators on studies of the relation between alcohol and breast cancer have criticized cohort studies that did not include negative mammograms in the cohort definition. By what definition of breast cancer might women with occult neoplasms at the beginning of observation be considered to be at risk during observation? By what definition would they not be at risk?

Why does standardization of compared risks or rates by definition eliminate confounding by the factor over which risks or rates are standardized?

Must the time that an individual contributes to a single category of person time be continuous, or can it be disjoint? Give an example.

Can events that preceded the time of observation in an open cohort study affect the categorization of an individual's person time under observation? Can they affect the categorization of a disease event?

## Case-Control Studies

What is the source population for a study of cases of myocardial infarction that are admitted to the emergency room of an urban hospital?

What is the source population for a study of deaths from myocardial infarction noted on death certificates held by the state of Massachusetts?

In Australia, persons eligible to vote are obliged by law to register with the election authorities, and the lists so created are a matter of public record. What is the importance of these lists for the conduct of case-control studies in Australia? Is there an argument for limiting the cases of case-control studies to eligible voters?

Under what circumstances might elderly nuns be an acceptable control series for a study in which the cases are sexually active young males?

Assume that case ascertainment involves a sophisticated diagnostic procedure that is not routinely available to persons who may have the disease under study. Describe the ways in which the results of a case-control study based on such ascertainment may be distorted. Would a cohort study using the same case ascertainment procedure be similarly affected?

# 13

# Statistical Terms and Concepts

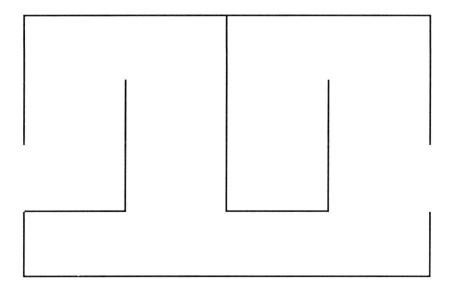

Although the concepts of contemporary epidemiology are not mathematical ones, there is no useful manipulation of the epidemiologic ideas that does not resort at some point to statistical inference. In this sense, epidemiology depends upon statistics in much the same way that physics depends on mathematics. What follows is not intended to substitute for a formal introduction to applied statistics, but is rather a sketch of a number of statistical terms used in epidemiology. The first section lists definitions of commonly used statistical terms; the second provides the rules by which the variance estimates appropriate to different sampling distributions can be combined to provide variance estimates for epidemiologic measures.

## Definitions

**Bias.** *The difference between the expected value of an estimator and the parameter whose value is being estimated is the bias of the estimator.*

**Binomial distribution** *is the probability distribution that describes the number of events observed in N opportunities to observe an event, when the probability of observing a single event at any opportunity is π, and is unaffected by the observation of an event at any other opportunity.*

$$\Pr(x \mid N) = \frac{N!}{x!(N-x)!} \pi^x (1 - \pi)^{N-x}$$

$$E(X) = \pi N$$

$$\mathrm{Var}(X) = N\pi(1 - \pi)$$

*The range of possible values for x is [0, N]. π is the binomial parameter.*

**Confidence interval.** *A confidence interval is a set of possible parameter values that are consistent with a body of observations in the sense that the p values for the data given any of the parameter values in the interval are greater than a specified amount, usually designated by α. The salient operational feature of a confidence interval is that it is calculated by a mechanism that has a priori a 1-α probability of including the true parameter value.*

**Estimate.** *An estimate is a realization of the estimator. The estimate is a function of the observed data.*

**Estimator.** *An estimator is a procedure for obtaining estimates. It is, equivalently, a random variable whose realization, the "estimate," will be taken as a measure of a parameter. The estimator is a function of random variables whose realizations are the data points being observed.*

**Expected value.** *The expected value of a random variable X is the average value that is observed in many repeated realizations of X. The expected value can be calculated from the probability distribution as*

$$E(X) = \sum x \Pr(x)$$

*where the summation is over all possible values of x.  It can be obtained from the probability density function as*

$$E(X) = \int x f(x) dx$$

*where the integration is over all possible values of x.  The expected value is a measure of the location of the probability distribution in the universe of possible values of x.*

**Hazard.** *The hazard is the limiting value of the probability of becoming an incident case per unit time among those at risk for becoming a case.*

**Mean square error.**  *The mean square error of an estimate is the expected value of the square of the deviation of the estimate from the parameter value of which it is an estimate.  The mean square error can be calculated from the probability distribution as*

$$MSE(\hat{\mu}) = \sum (\hat{\mu} - \mu)^2 Pr(\hat{\mu})$$

*and from the probability density function as*

$$MSE(\hat{\mu}) = \int (\hat{\mu} - \mu)^2 f(\hat{\mu}) dx$$

*where μ is the parameter and the symbol " ^ " indicates an estimate of the parameter. Mean square error is a measure of the dispersion of the realizations of the estimate around the parameter value. It is the sum of the variance and the square of the bias.*

$$MSE(\hat{\mu}) = Var(\hat{\mu}) + [Bias(\hat{\mu})]^2$$

**Normal distribution,** *also called the Gaussian distribution, is the probability density function that describes the distribution of realizations x of a continuous random variable X when the value x is the sum of a very large number of random variables whose probability distribution is arbitrary, but whose variances are of similar magnitude.*

$$f(X) = \frac{1}{\sqrt{2\pi}\sigma} \exp\left( -\frac{(x-\mu)^2}{2\sigma^2} \right)$$

$$E(X) = \mu$$

$$\mathrm{Var}(X) = \sigma^2$$

*The range of possible values for x is (-∞, +∞). μ and σ², the mean and variance, are the parameters of the Normal distribution. For the binomial and Poisson distributions, when the distribution of X is such that the probability of a realization at or near a limiting value is nearly zero, many of their properties can be approximated by considering them to be Normal distributions whose expected values and variances are derived from the corresponding binomial and Poisson definitions.*

**p value.** *The p value is the probability of occurrence of estimates that are as or more deviant from posited parameter values than the estimates actually obtained from a body of data. The p value is a function of observed data. It is the realization of a random variable whose distribution is uniform in the range [0,1] under posited parameter values, and whose distribution becomes non-uniform, with an increased density near zero, under specified kinds of deviation from the posited values.*

**Parameter.** *The terms other than those describing the circumstances of observation and the outcome in the formulaic presentation of a probability distribution are parameters. Parameters are not observable, but may be estimated from observations.*

**Poisson distribution** *is the probability distribution that describes the number of events observed in a block of person time when the expected number of events is directly proportional to the total person time of observation. Let θ be the expected number of events per unit of person time and λ = θP be the number of events expected in a block of person time of size P.*

$$\mathrm{Pr}(x) = \frac{\lambda^x e^{-\lambda}}{x!}$$

$$E(X) = \lambda$$

$$\mathrm{Var}(X) = \lambda$$

*The range of possible values for x is [0, ∞). λ is the Poisson parameter. If P is imagined as being composed of a very large number of discrete units of person time, so that the probability of an event in any person time unit is very small, then the probability distribution of the number of events in P may also be considered to be binomial, with N taken as the number of discrete person time units. All the formulas above are derivable from their binomial counterparts in the limiting case in which N approaches infinity, with P and λ constant.*

**Probability.** *The probability of observing a particular realization x of a random variable X is the fraction of instances in which x will be observed out of many repeated observations of X.*[70]

**Probability density.** *The probability density is the counterpart of the probability distribution for continuous random variables. The probability density is always described in formulaic terms as the "probability density function," designated by* f(x). *The probability of observing a realization x of X in the range [a,b] is*

$$\Pr(X \in [a,b]) = \int_{a}^{b} f(x)dx$$

**Probability distribution.** *The probability distribution of a random variable X is the collection of the probabilities of all possible realizations of X . A probability distribution can be characterized by listing or graphing the relation between x and* Pr(x), *or by presenting a formula that permits the calculation of* Pr(x) *for any value of x. The terms in such a formula other than x and terms describing the circumstances of observation are called "parameters." Probability distributions may also be characterized approximately by presenting their expected values and variances.*

**Standard deviation.** *The standard deviation of a random variable X is the square root of* Var(X).

**Standard error.** *The standard error of an estimate is the square root of the variance of the estimator.*

**Variance.** *The variance of a random variable is the expected value of the square of the deviation of x from the expected value of X. The variance can be calculated from the probability distribution as*

$$\mathrm{Var}(X) = \sum [x - \mathrm{E}(X)]^2 \Pr(x)$$

*and from the probability density function as*

---

70. See also Chapter 14.

$$Var(X) = \int [x - E(X)]^2 f(x) dx$$

*Variance is a measure of the dispersion of the realizations of X around the expected value.*

## Manipulating Variances

Most epidemiologic measures are composites of random variables and functions of random variables. In order to derive the variances of those measures, it is generally sufficient to apply one or both of the following rules.

**Variance of a sum**

$$Var(X_1 + X_2) = Var(X_1) + Var(X_2) + 2Cov(X_1, X_2)$$

**Variance of a function**

$$Var[g(X)] = \left(\frac{\partial g}{\partial X}\right)^2 Var(X)$$

where $Cov(X_1, X_2)$ is the covariance of $X_1$ and $X_2$. In the development below, the epidemiologic measures being summed will be taken to be independent, so that $Cov(X_1, X_2) = 0$.

**Table 13.1** Some useful derivatives

| Function | Derivative |
|:---:|:---:|
| $kX$ | $k$ |
| $\ln(X)$ | $X^{-1}$ |

If X is binomial and g(X) = X/N, that is to say if g(X) is a risk

$$Var\left(\frac{X}{N}\right) = \left(\frac{1}{N}\right)^2 N\pi(1 - \pi)$$

$$= \left(\frac{1}{N}\right)^2 \frac{N\pi(N - N\pi)}{N}$$

which can be estimated by substituting $x$ for $N\pi$

$$Var\left(\frac{X}{N}\right) \doteq \frac{x(N - x)}{N^3}$$

If X is Poisson and $g(X) = X/P$, that is to say if $g(X)$ is an incidence rate,

$$\operatorname{Var}\left(\frac{X}{P}\right) \doteq \left(\frac{1}{P}\right)^2 \lambda$$

which can be estimated by substituting $x$ for $\lambda$

$$\operatorname{Var}\left(\frac{X}{P}\right) = \frac{x}{P^2}$$

The variance of the natural logarithm of an incidence rate (the estimate of a hazard) is

$$\operatorname{Var}\left[\ln\left(\frac{X}{P}\right)\right] = \left(\frac{\lambda}{P}\right)^{-2} \frac{\lambda}{P^2}$$

which can be estimated as

$$\operatorname{Var}\left[\ln\left(\frac{X}{P}\right)\right] \doteq \frac{1}{x}$$

The variance of a rate difference (the estimate of a hazard difference) is

$$\operatorname{Var}\left(\frac{X_1}{P_1} - \frac{X_0}{P_0}\right) = \frac{\lambda_1}{P_1^2} + \frac{\lambda_0}{P_0^2}$$

which can be estimated as

$$\operatorname{Var}\left(\frac{X_1}{P_1} - \frac{X_0}{P_0}\right) \doteq \frac{x_1}{P_1^2} + \frac{x_0}{P_0^2}$$

The variance of the logarithm of a rate ratio (the estimate of a hazard ratio) is

$$\operatorname{Var}\left[\ln\left(\frac{X_1/P_1}{X_0/P_0}\right)\right] = \operatorname{Var}\left[\ln\left(\frac{X_1}{P_1}\right) - \ln\left(\frac{X_0}{P_0}\right)\right]$$

$$= \frac{1}{\lambda_1} + \frac{1}{\lambda_0}$$

which can be estimated as

$$\mathrm{Var}\left[\ln\left(\frac{X_1/P_1}{X_0/P_0}\right)\right] \doteq \frac{1}{x_1} + \frac{1}{x_0}$$

# 14

# Glossary of Epidemiologic Terms

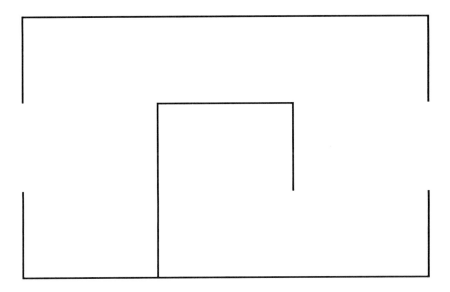

Definitions that occur in the text are repeated here for reference.

**Age effect.** *A change in disease incidence that is due to a biological concomitant of aging is an age effect.*

**Attack rate.** *The attack rate is the cumulative incidence of disease in persons who are exposed to an agent whose effect is shorter than the time of potential follow-up. The period of follow-up begins at the time of exposure and continues over a closed interval that allows the expression of all possible new cases attributable to the exposure.*

**Attributable risk.** See Incidence rate difference.

**Base population.** See Source population.

**Closed cohort.** *A closed cohort consists of individuals who are followed from a defined starting point to a defined end point. The membership of the group does not change, apart from mortality, from the beginning of observation to the end.*

**Cohort.** *Any group of individuals whose disease or mortality is measured over time is a cohort.*

**Cohort effect.** *Changes in disease frequency that are shared by all members of a group who entered follow-up at common time constitute a cohort effect.*

**Confounding.** *When imbalances in the composition of compared groups give rise to an expected value of a comparative measure that differs from the effect of the factor that defines the groups, the crude estimate of the effect of that factor is said to be confounded.*

**Controls.** *The controls in a case-control study are a group of persons whose exposure status collectively provides information about the distribution of exposure in the persons or person time giving rise to the cases.*

**Cumulative exposure.** *The cumulative exposure from time $t_0$ to time $t_1$ for an individual is the summation of all exposures endured from $t_0$ up until $t_1$.*

**Cumulative incidence.** *The cumulative incidence from time $t_0$ to time $t_1$ for event $X$ is the prevalence of "history of $X$" at time $t_1$ among all those persons who began observation at time $t_0$ and did not possess a "history of $X$" at time $t_0$.*

**Duration.** *The duration of an illness is the length of the time interval that elapses from first manifestation of disease until complete resolution. For an irreversible disease process, duration is the length of the interval from first manifestation to death.*

**Dynamic cohort.** See Open cohort.

**Etiologic fraction.** See Relative excess incidence.

**Exposure odds.** *The number of exposed persons divided by the number of unexposed persons in a group yields the exposure odds. The exposure odds in a pool of person time are obtained by dividing the amount of exposed person-time by the amount of unexposed person-time.*

**Fixed cohort.** See Closed cohort.

**Hazard.** *The hazard is the limiting value of the probability of becoming an incident case per unit time among those at risk for becoming a case.*

**Immortal person-time.** *The experience of study subjects that is event-free by definition is immortal person-time.*

**Inception cohort.** *The persons who are under observation at the beginning of an exposure that defines cohort membership are termed an inception cohort.*

**Incidence density.** See Incidence rate.

**Incidence proportion.** See Cumulative incidence.

**Incidence rate.** *The incidence rate of an event in a block of person time is the number of events observed divided by the amount of person time observed.*

**Incidence rate difference.** *The incidence rate difference is the difference between the incidence in an exposed population and that in an unexposed population.*

**Incidence rate ratio.** *The incidence rate ratio is the ratio of the incidence rate in an exposed population to that in an unexposed population.*

**Incident.** *A case of disease is said to be "incident" at the moment at which the disease manifests signs or symptoms. Incident cases are newly occurring cases.*

**Induction period.** *The induction period is the time required for the effects of a specific exposure to become manifest.*

**Latency.** *The time interval during which a disease is latent. Also, in occupational epidemiology, the interval from first exposure to observation.*

**Latent.** *A disease that is present but not symptomatic is latent.*

**Nested** *describes a case-control study for which the source population is one whose person time (open cohort) or persons (closed cohort) has been previously identified and enumerated for research purposes.*

**Open cohort.** *An open cohort is a cohort whose composition changes with the passage of time.*

**Period effect.** *Changes in disease frequency that are specific to a calendar time are collectively termed a period effect.*

**Person time** *is the time during which a single individual meets all the definitions for inclusion in a study, and during which any disease event occurring in the individual would be known. The person time of observation in a population is the sum of the person times contributed by all the members of the population.*

**Population attributable risk.** See Population rate difference.

**Population rate difference.** *The difference between an incidence rate in a population comprising both exposed and unexposed persons and the rate in a population comprising unexposed persons alone is the population rate difference.*

**Prevalence.** *The prevalence of a characteristic in a population is the fraction of individuals in the population who possess the characteristic.*

**Probability** *is a characteristic of the physical processes that give rise to observable events, and represents the limiting value that would be observed for an cumulative incidence or a prevalence as larger and larger numbers of individuals came under scrutiny.*[71]

**Prospective.** *A prospective study is one in which the disease events under study occur after the protocol for data collection has been implemented.*

---

71. See also Chapter 13.

**Relative excess incidence.** *The relative excess incidence is the fraction of the disease burden among exposed that would not have occurred if the exposed had experienced the same incidence rate as the unexposed.*

**Residual effect.** *The changes in disease incidence that are attributable to an exposure are said to be the residual effect of that exposure if they are observable after the exposure has ceased.*

**Retrospective.** *A retrospective study is one in which the protocol is implemented after the disease events have occurred.*

**Risk.** See Probability.

**Sampling.** *The process of selecting a study population from a source population, with the goal of learning about characteristics of the source population, is known as sampling.*

**Source population.** *The individuals about whose experience or condition a study yields data are the source population. A source population is defined by the identity of the individuals whom it comprises and by the time periods during which each individual is considered to be a member.*

**Standard.** *The set of weights used for standardization is the standard. These weights sum to 1.*

**Standardization.** *Standardized measures are formed from a series of individual measures by taking a weighted average of the individual values.*

**Study population.** *The study population is the group of individuals that an investigator observes.*

**Survival** *is the complement of disease occurrence over a time interval. The observed survival is 1 minus the cumulative incidence of disease.*

**Survivor cohort.** *The persons who remain under observation at some point after the beginning of an exposure that defines cohort membership are a survivor cohort.*

# Acknowledgements

While writing the various chapters of this book, I have been supported by the Burroughs-Wellcome Fund, the Carnegie Mellon Fund, the International Agency for Research on Cancer, and the National Cancer Institute. The chapters on disease frequency, comparisons, and sampling strategies are based on texts written for the Eastern Cooperative Oncology Group, at Marvin Zelen's suggestion. Earlier versions of the chapters on cohort and case-control studies were written for David Zaridze, for inclusion in a Russian textbook of cancer epidemiology. The chapter on confounding is drawn almost verbatim from work carried out with Stephan Lanes. The chapter on the reporting of epidemiologic studies appeared in a somewhat different form in the American Journal of Public Health. Jacques Dunnigan suggested the topic of risk perception and communication and provided a forum for me to air these ideas. All of the texts have benefited greatly from the criticisms and suggestion of students at the Harvard School of Public Health and the Harvard Medical School. Dimitrios Trichopoulos and Chung-Cheng Hsieh kindly pointed out many errors of grammar, notation, and logic, which I have corrected. Sander Greenland has held me to a higher standard than has any other critic; this book owes much that is consistent and well-said to him.

My own teacher's voices hum in the back of my thoughts when I try to lay out an introductory essay. If Ken Rothman, Hershel Jick, and Olli Miettinen see their words here, I trust that they will understand the imitation as thanks.

# Index

Bold type indicates definitions. Definitions in the main text are embedded within more extensive discussions, which are not separately listed below.

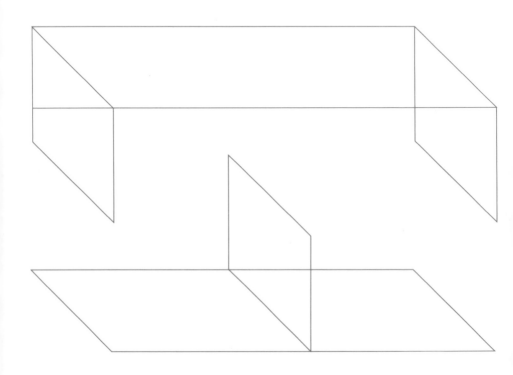

*ERI*

*Epidemiology Resources Inc.*

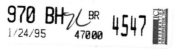

ISBN 0-917227-07-7